Doctors Talking with Patients/Patients Talking with Doctors

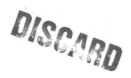

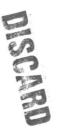

Doctors Talking with Patients/Patients Talking with Doctors

IMPROVING COMMUNICATION IN MEDICAL VISITS

SECOND EDITION

DEBRA L. ROTER & JUDITH A. HALL

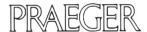
PRAEGER

Westport, Connecticut
London

Library of Congress Cataloging-in-Publication Data

Roter, Debra.
  Doctors talking with patients/patients talking with doctors : improving
communication in medical visits / Debra L. Roter and Judith A. Hall. — 2nd ed.
     p. ; cm.
  Includes bibliographical references and index.
  ISBN 0-275-99014-1 (alk. paper) — ISBN 0-275-99017-6 (pbk : alk. paper)
  1. Physician and patient. 2. Communication in medicine. I. Hall, Judith A.
II. Title.
  [DNLM: 1. Communication. 2. Office Visits. 3. Physician-Patient
Relations. W 62 R843d 2006]
  R727.3.R68 2006
  610.69'6—dc22   2006020999

British Library Cataloguing in Publication Data is available.

Library of Congress Catalog Card Number: 2006020999
ISBN: 0-275-99014-1 (cloth)
        0-275-99017-6 (pbk.)

First published in 2006

Praeger Publishers, 88 Post Road West, Westport, CT 06881
An imprint of Greenwood Publishing Group, Inc.
www.praeger.com

Printed in the United States of America

The paper used in this book complies with the
Permanent Paper Standard issued by the National
Information Standards Organization (Z39.48-1984).

10   9   8   7   6   5   4   3   2   1

We dedicate this book to our spouses, Eric Waller and Fred Gordon, and our children: Saul, Ben, and Annie Rose, and Jacob, Rebecca, and Sarah. And, we dedicate this book to one another and the gifts of work, inspiration, passion, humor, and fun that we have had the good fortune to share.

Contents

Tables

Preface to the Second Edition

Since the publication of the first edition of this book almost 15 years ago, medicine has undergone a transformation. Unlike the earlier revolutions in medicine, spurred by advances in technology and pharmacology, the current transformation has been driven by a political, professional, and scientific dialogue on health care quality, medical errors, health care financing, and health care delivery systems. In the past several years, three Institute of Medicine reports have included a primary focus on the nature and quality of medical communication (Institute of Medicine, 1999, 2001, 2003). Moreover, health communication objectives are included in the surgeon general's Healthy People 2010 objectives for the nation (U.S. Department of Health and Human Services, 1999). Related to these national reports, unprecedented reforms in medical education have been promulgated by the profession's accrediting and credentialing bodies. Beginning in 2002, the American Association of Medical Colleges (AAMC) and the American College of Graduate Medical Education (ACGME) added competency requirements for graduates in six core skills, including interpersonal communication. The significance of these changes has reverberated across the medical education spectrum; virtually every training institution in the country has undertaken a review of its medical curriculum and the way it trains physicians.

These sweeping reforms have been accompanied by an exponential growth in research addressing the nature, dynamics, contexts, and consequences of the medical dialogue. It is with great delight and excitement that we have undertaken the task of preparing a second edition of our book.

THE STRUCTURE OF THIS BOOK AND REVISIONS TO THE SECOND EDITION

All chapters have been updated with references to current literature, some sections have been expanded to include new areas of inquiry, and new chapters have been added to this book to accommodate the much richer literature that now exists in this area. This book is divided into three parts. Part I is descriptive in nature and is designed to reflect what is known about the effect of sociodemographic and contextual variables on how doctors and patients typically behave; it also addresses some of the methodological issues related to how we know this, from a variety of vantage points. Part II describes what usually happens in medical visits, to provide the reader with insight into how predictable medical visits really are, but it also describes what outcomes can be expected and how both the process and the result might be improved. Part III discusses in more depth some of the valuable outcomes that might follow from improved doctor-patient talk.

Chapter 1 begins with a broad overview of the significance of talk to the doctor-patient relationship and the therapeutic process. The significance of talk is discussed within the context of eight communication-transforming principles that are designed to demonstrate not only the critical role talk plays in the medical care process, but also our conviction that the talk of the visit can be changed for the better. The implications of transformed talk are pivotal to the fundamental way medicine is practiced. It is the first step to a transformed medical model that is relationship-centered and optimally effective. We conclude this chapter by adding a final communication-transforming principle, one that captures the contribution of the doctor-patient relationship itself to the processes and outcomes of care.

The second chapter explores the ideal form of the doctor-patient relationship, as presented through model prototypes. The relationship models explore the unstated ground rules for routine exchanges and provide insight into the rich diversity of forms that relationships may take. These forms range from relationships in which paternalism predominates to collaborative partnerships, with much variation in between. The chapter focuses on the varying nature of talk, which, during the medical visit, supports and molds the form that the doctor-patient relationship will take. Following the discussion of relationship prototypes, a third chapter, on theoretical and methodological issues in studying medical communication, has been added. This chapter provides a foundation for evaluating the field in terms of its theoretical relevance and methodological utility; it also provides a framework through which the many research findings and innovations presented throughout the remainder of this book may be understood.

Many factors contribute to how an individual doctor or patient may behave during the medical visit. Some of these factors are highly individual, like personality traits and prior experiences—but many factors are not. Sociodemographic characteristics, for instance, are quite predictive of both patient and physician behaviors. Chapters 4–6 address both social and personal characteristics that affect patient and provider behavior. For patients, a rich literature is reviewed in Chapter 4, documenting the important ways talk is influenced by such sociodemographic variables as age, race, gender, education, and social class. These areas of discussion have been expanded in several ways. An expanded section has been added that explores the implications of how patient age affects visit dynamics; this section includes a discussion of the increasing likelihood of a visit companion, often a spouse or adult child, in geriatric medical visits. We have also expanded our earlier discussion of education to include a discussion of the role of health literacy in the communication dynamics of medical visits. We have also followed several lines of new, and potentially exciting, research (identified in the first edition) related to other patient characteristics. For instance, we discussed the effects of the patient's health status on the medical dialogue and noted that, while it appeared to be important, there were few published studies on the subject. Similarly, we noted, with great theoretical interest, the role that "liking" may play in the doctor-patient relationship, raising such questions as which patients and physicians are liked more than others, how accurate each may be in predicting the degree to which he or she is liked by the other, and how mutual their liking may be. We have pursued these lines of inquiry over the years, and the second edition presents new sections within Chapter 4 that are devoted to recent studies in each of these areas.

The literature is generally less rich in the description of physician characteristics associated with visit talk and the care given to patients than it is in its descriptions of patients. However, many more studies addressing the influence of physician characteristics and attributes in relation to physician communication style have been conducted over the past decade. For example, the current literature is beginning to address the influence of physician race and ethnicity on the physician's interpersonal communication with patients. Because there were virtually no studies in this area when the first edition was written, we have added several new sections to Chapter 5 that are devoted to aspects of this topic. Other physician characteristics, including personality and attitudes toward the psychological component of medical problems, may also be associated with patient care and are discussed in this chapter, as well.

The change in this area that is most notable is the study of physician gender. Because this is an area in which we have conducted much of our own research, and which we still find to be fascinating, we have added a chapter on this subject (Chapter 6). In Chapter 6, we describe how a physician's gender affects his or her communication with patients, as well as how a physician's gender influences the way in which his or her patients communicate.

Part II of this book describes what usually happens during medical visits. This bird's-eye view is intended to provide the reader with insight into how predictable medical visits really are and how both the process and the result might be improved through interventions. In Chapter 7, we offer an anatomical guide, of sorts, to the medical interview, describing its structure, function, content, and duration. The information here should be both familiar (as you will no doubt recognize from the visits you have had) and surprising because of how standardized most exchanges are. An additional section has been added to this chapter, providing international comparisons to the typical U.S. primary care medical visits.

Not all talk that occurs during the medical visit is of equal importance to the care process. In Chapter 8, the particularly critical role of information exchange is examined. The two-way flow of information in medical encounters and its role in establishing the basis for mutual understanding are explored. Within this context, inquiry into the dynamics of patient decision making and the facilitative role of physicians in those decisions has been growing. Consequently, a new section, devoted to the area of patient involvement in medical decision making, has been added.

The third and final part of this book is devoted in more depth to the consequences and future of doctor-patient talk. Chapter 9 discusses patient satisfaction with care, compliance with medical recommendations, functional status, quality of life, and morbidity in relation to variations in the nature of medical visit talk. Chapter 10 demonstrates the surprising ease with which important improvements in the process and outcome of care can be achieved through experimental interventions. Finally, in light of 15 years' hindsight, we present an endnote to the book in which we revisit the speculations presented in the first edition.

As we hope it is evident in the pages of this book, we believe there are important ways in which the exchanges of doctors and patients can be improved, for the benefit of both. In emphasizing the doctor-patient relationship, we do not imply, of course, that all the woes of the medical system can be traced to that source. In the United States, ever-rising costs of health care and prescription medications are a terrible burden to the economy, and millions of citizens cannot afford proper medical care. These problems, among many others, cannot be solved by studying what happens within the four walls of a doctor's office.

But what happens within those walls is extremely important. The words and gestures, the emotions felt and communicated, the decisions, the attitudes, and the presumptions made by both sides are key elements of the medical experience. Encounters with doctors are highly charged—often comforting and rewarding, but sometimes upsetting and disappointing. Patients often remember, word for word, their exchanges with their doctors, and these exchanges are frequently recited for family members and friends and played back over and over in the patient's mind. For some people, the words comprising the remembered dialogue of a past medical visit take on the full significance of a life event, creating distress anew in each repetition—or providing comfort and reassurance.

The significance of doctor-patient communication goes far beyond momentary hopes and disappointments; years of research now prove that these exchanges have far-reaching impacts on the lives of patients. A patient's interest in the health care process, willingness to visit doctors, adherence to health care goals, knowledge about his or her medical condition(s), and health itself can be traced to the character of these exchanges.

Like many who study health and illness and the process of medical care, we believe that medical care is a social process, as well as a technical one. In other words, medical care involves more than accurate diagnoses and correct recommendations for treatment. Social factors precede diagnoses, for they are involved in the very experience and definition of illness and the willingness to seek care. Social and psychological processes imbue every event and decision in medical care. Medicine is not a narrowly defined technical enterprise, no matter how sophisticated the technologies become. Many doctors and patients undoubtedly recognize how profoundly social the process of medical care is, but probably few, in either group, are aware of how well developed our scientific knowledge of that process is. In writing this book, we hope to introduce this important body of research to those who will profit from it most—the doctors and patients who have been its subject.

Our focus in writing this book is, as the title suggests, talk. The term *talk* is meant broadly, to include all of the face-to-face communications, including nonverbal ones, that are exchanged between doctors and patients. In writing about the process of care, we use the vernacular word *doctor* to refer to a person with an M.D. or D.O. degree. In this book, the word *physician* is interchangeable with the word *doctor.* We sometimes also refer to providers and practitioners, terms that include doctors and other professionals who provide health care, such as nurses, nurse practitioners, and physicians' assistants.

This book is not an attack on doctors, nor an attack on patients, nor an attack on the institutions within which doctors and patients interact. However, doctors and patients, alike, can work to understand the shortcomings in their relationships, and together they can work to correct them. If we take it as our job to communicate these shortcomings and suggest avenues of improvement, we do so in the hope of enhancing the medical experience for *both* doctors and patients. Underlying the work presented in this book is the confidence that doctors and patients can change the nature of their interactions. If we accomplish nothing else, we hope to encourage doctors and patients to reflect on the possibility of eliciting new repertoires of responses from one another. This requires gaining insight into how each typically behaves, developing an agenda for what an improved relationship would look like, and recognizing that each person tends to act in a manner consistent with the other's expectations. Our goal is to convey enough knowledge to convince doctors and patients of the necessity for change, and to promote a sense of empowerment in them.

Part I

The Nature of the
Doctor-Patient Relationship

1

The Significance of Talk

This book is about doctors and patients and what goes on between them in medical visits. Most of what occurs is talk. By talk we mean what is said in the verbal sense—the words that are used, the facts exchanged, the advice given, and the social amenities that tie the conversation together. But we also mean communication beyond words, the whole repertoire of nonverbal expressions and cues within which verbal transactions are embedded. The smiles and head nods of agreement, the grimaces of pain, the high-pitched voice of anxiety, and the various subtle cues indicative of interpersonal dominance (to give some examples); all of these nonverbal expressions give context and enhanced meaning to the words spoken.

Despite its central role, awareness of the nature of this talk is often not very high. This occurs for several reasons. The conversation often feels very routine, as when the doctor and patient exchange a perfunctory "hi-how-are-you-I'm-fine" greeting. The exchanges are often highly scripted and do not leave many options (such as the question-answer routine of a medical history taking). And, much of the nonverbal behavior that people engage in and respond to remains below the threshold of awareness. There are exceptions, of course. A doctor might give careful thought to which questions to ask and how to phrase them, or a doctor might take conscious note of a look of perplexity or discomfort on the patient's face. A patient might phrase a question ahead of time, lament oversights in descriptions of symptoms, or notice that the doctor seemed to be in a hurry. But generally the exchange is taken for granted, with the participants having little sense that they choose how it develops, that it can be different than it typically is, and that it has a profound impact not just on the doctor-patient relationship but also on the outcomes of care. Very often, awareness of the communication process occurs only after there has been a breakdown in communication, leading one or both of the parties to feel confused, disappointed, frustrated, or angry.

The perspective of this book is that talk is the one of the two fundamental ingredients of medical care. The other fundamental ingredient is the expert knowledge that both participants bring to their encounter: the doctor is an expert on diagnoses, treatments, and the like, and the patient is an expert on his or her own history, values, intuitions, and experience. Talk is certainly the fundamental instrument by which the doctor-patient relationship is crafted and by which therapeutic goals are achieved. Though physicians conduct physical exams and use blood tests, X-rays, medications, and other tools to achieve therapeutic goals, the value of these activities is limited without the talk that organizes the history and symptoms and puts them in a meaningful context for both the patient and the physician.

Our high regard for the role of talk is far from universally accepted. Historians of modern medicine have tracked the changing patterns of medical practice to reveal a fundamental shift in the centrality of talk to the care process. In his study of the history of doctors and patients, Edward Shorter (1985) identified the post–World War II era as a pivotal time for modern medicine. The discovery of sulfa drugs in the 1930s, and, later, penicillin in the 1940s, transformed the practice of medicine. The transformation was, however, not so much in the prescription of these drugs, but in their impact on medical training. The drug revolution led medicine to the chemistry-oriented sciences of biochemistry, microbiology, pharmacology, immunology, and genetics; this led medicine toward a mainly organic picture of disease, as something to be combated with drugs. The battle lines were drawn between the doctor and the aberrant molecules, and the patient was often left on the sidelines. Thus, the world saw the birth of the "biomedical" model of disease and medicine's diminished interest in the patient's experience of illness.

Shorter (1985) maintained that this depersonalization of medicine was downgrading the importance of history taking and performing physical exams in lieu of more structured data collection and the interpretation of laboratory data. It is not coincidental that the practice of interviewing patients from a written outline designed around a series of yes-no questions began during this time. The patient's talk was largely curtailed by these changes and was restricted to answering the questions asked. One important effect of these changes was to recast the medical interview as wholly scientific and objective.

It can be further argued that the scientific recasting of the medical dialogue contributed to a loss of physician confidence in the significance of any but the most explicit hypothesis-driven exchanges and quantified findings. Using the notions of high- and low-context communication cultures as articulated by anthropologist Edward T. Hall, medicine can be seen as having undergone a shift from a high- to low-context communication endeavor (E. T. Hall, 1976). High-context communication depends on sensitivity to nonverbal behaviors and environmental cues to decipher meaning, while low-context exchanges are more verbally explicit with little reliance on the unstated or nuanced. One manifestation of this shift in medicine is the diminished attention paid to emotion and its role in the care process. It is our thesis that the doctor-patient relationship is an intrinsically high-context phenomenon, within which the communication of expert knowledge and emotions are central. Both the physician and the patient are experts, though the domains of their expertise are typically very different. Physicians are experts in the technical and cognitive ways that are emphasized in their training. Patients are experts in their own histories, experiences of illness, personalities, lifestyles, life settings, values, and expectations.

In part, the focus on scientific objectivity reflects a widespread characterization of medicine as taking place in a context of potential death, disability, trauma, pain, and uncertainty. Patients are thought to defend themselves against feelings of overwhelming complexity, demoralization, and helplessness by recourse to idealization or denigration of the physician. Physicians, on the other hand, also need to protect themselves from feelings of grief and helplessness made worse by an overriding sense of their ever-present potential for making a fatal error (Hilfiker, 1985). In this context of heightened emotions and defensive responses, the stereotypical encounter is characterized as a retreat from rational (logical) communication on the part of the patient, and a retreat to pure rationalism (to the "science" of medicine) on the part of the physician.

But a necessary perspective on this quite dramatic portrait is gained by recognizing that, in fact, most of the illnesses seen in medical encounters are not of the extreme kind. Clinically urgent and very frightening diseases are very much the exception in everyday medical practice. Moreover, even the most severe illnesses tend to lead to routine, maintenance-centered encounters over time (Tuckett, Boulton, Olson, & Williams, 1985). Despite a reality reflecting a rather nondramatic routine, the illusion of drama remains and subverts the talk that explores the everyday matters of concern.

The denigration of talk between doctors and patients acts to restrict the many therapeutic purposes it serves. For the patient, the talk of the visit gives meaning and legitimacy to feelings of fear and physical discomfort; just naming a medical condition helps enormously in this regard. Through talk, doctors and patients express who they are, what they expect of each other, and what kind of relationship they have. And talk has powerful consequences. A patient's very motivation to get well can be seen as springing from the quality of exchange with his or her doctor. Physicians need talk as well. Diagnoses can be extremely misguided without adequate talk. Without talk, patient and doctor may never even reach a common understanding of the purpose of the medical visit.

Because of deficiencies in talk, the routine medical visit does not nearly reach its therapeutic potential. Diagnosis could be more accurate, medical intervention more effective, recovery more speedy, realization of quality of life more complete, and satisfaction for both doctor and patient more likely. What is wrong is not simply a matter of fault. As we will explore in this book, the patient-physician relationship is burdened on both sides by deep-seated stereotypes and traditions. Although it is debatable whether the relationship ever really served its patients and practitioners as well as nostalgic recollections of the "good old days" maintain, there is little doubt that it is less than perfectly suited to contemporary needs. The challenge is to understand better and then reshape the relationship so that it may indeed achieve its healing potential.

Our purpose in writing this book is to demonstrate that the talk of the medical visit can be changed for the better and that this in itself can transform the way in which medicine is practiced. The positive changes advocated here can be summarized in eight communication-transforming principles: (1) communication should serve the patient's need to tell the story of his or her illness and the doctor's need to hear it; (2) communication should reflect the special expertise and insight that the patient has into his or her physical state and well being; (3) communication should reflect and respect the relationship between a patient's mental state and his or her physical experience of illness; (4) communication should maximize the usefulness of the physician's expertise; (5) communication should acknowledge and attend to the emotional content of the communication; (6) communication should openly reflect the principle of reciprocity, in which the fulfillment of expectations is negotiated; (7) communication should help participants overcome stereotyped roles and expectations so that both participants in the medical encounter gain a sense of power and the freedom to change; and (8) communication should facilitate the development of the doctor-patient relationship because the relationship itself has the power to shape the processes and outcomes of care.

These communication principles will be described in some detail in the remainder of this chapter and will provide the themes that run through the entire book. They are critical for a transformed medical practice and a better model of doctor-patient communication.

THE IMPORTANCE OF TELLING THE STORY

The doctor-patient relationship is different from other relationships. People expect the doctor to know them in a fundamental and intimate way, and doctors need to know their patients in order to truly care and cure. This is the first communication-transforming principle: *Communication should serve the patient's need to tell the story of his or her illness and the doctor's need to hear it.* Telling the story is the method by which the meaning of the illness and the meaning of the disease are integrated and interpreted by both doctor and patient.

Patients need to feel that their doctors take a personal interest in them as individuals, like them, are concerned and committed to their welfare, and will consequently take pains to do a good job. The fulfillment of the basic need to feel known and understood begins with the telling of the patient's story. Telling one's story can also be therapeutic in its own right because it provides a cathartic release and the opportunity for insight and perspective. For physicians, the patient's story provides the context for the clinical insight necessary for understanding and interpreting the many symptoms and clues the patient provides.

The arithmetic of each physician having an average of 2,500 patients does not equal the experience of each of those 2,500 patients with his or her doctor. Each patient expects that treatment will be uniquely suited to his or her individual needs, but the patient must express these needs within the constraints of short appointment blocks scheduled several times throughout the year. It is in this context that patients attempt to establish their unique identities—where patients search for the opportunity to tell their stories and to experience the feeling that their stories are heard.

But the telling is not so easy. Stories may not be told because patients fear that the stories do not meet the standards of life-and-death intensity the patients assume their doctors demand. This is unfortunate—especially so because the patient's assumption that the doctor is not interested or that the story is unimportant is infrequently addressed in an explicit manner. If the doctor does not facilitate the story telling—if the patient is not encouraged to go on—the patient very often will not.

Facilitating the story-telling process is best accomplished when there are no strict parameters limiting or defining the patient's response. The patient's story is not limited to the first-presenting problem. Patients often state a medical complaint as a "ticket of entry" to medical care, even though the primary and most pressing concern may be unrelated to this complaint.

A study focusing on the first 90 seconds of the medical visit found that the patient's response to the physician's opening question was completed in only 23% of the visits studied. In 69% of the visits, the physician interrupted the patient's opening statement, after an average of only 15 seconds, to follow up on a stated problem. In only one of these visits was the patient given the opportunity to return to, and complete, the opening statement. For those 30% of patients who were allowed to continue, none of their statements took more than 2.5 minutes (Beckman & Frankel, 1984). Moreover, analysis of the concerns raised by patients throughout the visit showed that the first named concern was no more clinically significant than concerns that were expressed later. However, later concerns tended to be raised in a haphazard manner and they received inconsistent attention from the physician. A replication of this study some 15 years later (Marvel, Epstein, Flowers, & Beckman, 1999) found little had changed in physicians' attention to their patients' agenda; patients' initial statements of concern were completed in only 28% of interviews, and their opening statements were redirected after an average of 23 seconds.

Because of embarrassment, fear of appearing foolish, or real anxiety about the possible meaning of symptoms, patients' "secondary" concerns are often hidden beneath the surface of "more legitimate" medical complaints. The unstated concerns have been referred to as the patient's hidden agenda, and it is especially dreaded by physicians when it surfaces as the patient is leaving, as an aside (Stoeckle & Barsky, 1981). The dreaded doorway question, "By the way, doctor, I have chest tightness (a lump in my breast, swelling in my legs, some problems remembering things, etc.), but that's nothing to worry about, right?" can necessitate a time-consuming extension of the medical visit. One study estimated that 20% of routine primary care visits have a new problem introduced during the visit's closing minutes (J. White, Levinson, & Roter, 1994). The Marvel et al. (1999) study that was mentioned earlier found that the raising of concerns late in the visit was associated with failures to solicit the patient's agenda during the visit opening. The researchers found that patients were nearly twice as likely to introduce new concerns after the history segment was complete if the physician had not attempted to solicit the patient's agenda during the visit opening.

Another element of story telling is an exploration of the significance and impact of the illness or medical problem for the patient. How patients understand their diseases and the attributions the patients make are extremely important in understanding their reactions and fears. Inordinate distress, for example, may stem more from patients' beliefs about what is wrong than from the disease itself. Most patients hold some kind of theory about the specific causative factor for their symptoms or conditions. Knowledge of a patient's attribution can be helpful, in that it may reveal some of the patient's personal and emotional experiences, which in fact may be what are prompting the visit. However, a patient may be reluctant at first to volunteer his or her thoughts, for fear of appearing ignorant or foolish. The patient may have an incorrect biomechanical explanation for the symptoms and may need education and explanation, or the patient may subscribe to religious or cultural beliefs that are at odds with a "scientific explanation."

Once these beliefs are out in the open, then some middle ground and accommodation may be reached.

Most patients also have particular expectations in mind when they visit the doctor, although they may be reluctant to make these known directly. Expectations may be for particular treatment (drugs or tests), administrative help, or, most commonly, simply for a better understanding of the etiology, diagnosis, prognosis, or treatment of the condition and how these relate to the patient's prior experiences or the experiences of others they know.

All of these things, feeling known and understood, having the opportunity for catharsis, insight, and perspective, as well as conveying the life context of the illness, its meaning, interpretation, and the patient's expectations for care, are part of the story the patient tells.

PATIENTS AS EXPERTS

This brings us to a second communication-transforming principle: *The patient should be considered an "expert" in his or her own right and therefore to have unique perspectives and valuable insights into his or her physical state, functional status, and quality of life.* In studies of over 23,000 people (Idler & Kasl, 1991), investigators have concluded that a simple self-evaluation of health—the answer to the question, "At the present time, how would you rate your health?"—provides strong clues to patient survival over periods as long as seventeen years. Furthermore, people's self-evaluations of health were stronger predictors of death than "objective" indicators of health, including detailed physical exams and batteries of tests. Professionals' recognition of the importance of patients' self-ratings of health makes an interesting story.

The first studies performed in this area were done in an attempt to validate the "subjective" patient ratings of the patient's own health against the gold-standard of physicians' "objective" ratings. The assumption was that a physician's insight into the health of an individual was more clinically accurate than the individual's own evaluation. After all, physicians are trained to make health assessments and have a wide array of sophisticated technology at their disposal. However, since self-evaluations were so frequently asked for in health surveys, there was some interest in determining how valid they were—that is, how closely they matched the physicians' evaluations.

The predominant findings showed that self-ratings and physicians' ratings of an individual's health were similar in the majority of cases; however, the relationship was far from perfect, and significant differences were quite common. Discrepancies in patient and physician ratings were most often the result of patient "health optimism." Patients were two to three times more likely to rate their health better than their physicians rated it. When the opposite was the case, however, and patients' self-ratings of health were poor, researchers found an increased likelihood of impending death. Elderly patients in the Yale Health and Aging Project (Idler & Kasl, 1991) who self-rated their health as poor were three to six times (females and males, respectively) more likely to die within the four-year follow-up period than those who rated their health as excellent. This risk remained even when a host of "objective" factors, such as the number of health problems, disabilities, and health risk factors were taken into account. It appears that self-rated health has a unique, predictive, and largely unexplained relationship with death and survival; it also appears that this relationship is more predictive than any prognosis a doctor can provide.

Why would self-evaluations of present health predict future mortality so well, and better than physician assessments? No one really knows. The authors of the Yale Health and Aging Project suggested two alternative explanations. First, it is possible that there is a direct effect of health optimism or pessimism on subsequent health. Optimism may lead to a denial of vulnerability, leading to a healthier sense of self; if one thinks of oneself as healthy, acts and looks healthy, and is perceived by others as healthy, then one may indeed become healthy. Or, optimism can act indirectly to enhance health by encouraging healthy actions. Since optimists tend to anticipate positive outcomes for their efforts and may be less discouraged by setbacks, they may be more inclined to undertake lifestyle changes and make health-promoting choices about diet and other aspects of lifestyle. An interesting study by de Ridder and colleagues suggests that it is the latter that may be the more likely explanation (de Ridder, Fournier, & Bensing, 2004). Based on their study of chronically ill patients, the authors concluded that optimistic patients did not have unrealistic perceptions of their health status, but that they were more likely to engage in self-care behavior. Moreover, increased engagement in self-care led to better physical functioning 6 months later.

There is also the possibility that self-evaluations reflect a calculation of life expectancy based on a broad range of information that is known only to the individual. This might include such "objective" things as the patient's chronic disease history and the longevity of the patient's parents and grandparents, or more "subjective" feelings, such as the patient's energy and well-being.

Another explanation for the predictive validity of self-evaluations is related to judgments of quality of life. Physicians tend to associate general health ratings with the number and severity of chronic conditions, irrespective of the effect of these conditions on the patient's quality of life. However, the impact of disabilities associated with health conditions is highly variable and contingent not only on the individuals themselves, but on their social networks and resources. These factors include family members, friends, and neighbors who supply help in its many forms, through social contact, direct services, money, and emotional support to enhance an individual's ability to cope with and adapt to physical, social, and environmental challenges. The process of adaptation reflects a daily experience of quality of life. Self-evaluations of health are largely associated with this aspect of living, which is not necessarily known or fully appreciated by physicians, or by family and friends, for that matter.

Indeed, it has been found that patients' and physicians' understandings of "overall health" differ in basic meaning, with physicians relying on medical data, while patients draw on the physical, functional, social, and emotional aspects of their health (J. A. Hall, Epstein, & McNeil, 1989; Martin, Gilson, Bergner, Bobbitt, Pollard, Conn, & Cole, 1976). In the study performed by Hall and colleagues, the patients' ratings were related to their functional abilities (such as the ability to walk without a cane or dress without help), their emotional distress, and the number of different medical diagnoses appearing in their medical charts. It seems the patients appropriately considered overall health to be a broad notion that covered three distinct ways of being "healthy." The doctors' ratings, on the other hand, were related mainly to the number of diagnoses the patient had—a much narrower frame of reference. The doctors' understanding of overall health, therefore, seemed constrained by the biomedical point of view (health as defined by medical words in the chart) and not informed by the state of health as the patient experienced it.

Other research on reports of health by patients versus doctors, nurses, or family members also shows disparities between points of view, and the disparities take a similar form. Hospitalized patients have reported themselves as functioning better than their nurses report; elderly people have reported themselves to be less emotionally distressed than a proxy respondent (usually a family member) reports; patients have reported themselves to be less depressed and more physically healthy than their doctors say they are (Epstein, Hall, Tognetti, Son, & Conant, 1989; J. A. Hall, Stein, Roter, & Rieser, 1999; Rubenstein, Schairer, Wieland, & Kane, 1984; Yager & Linn, 1981). As in the Idler and Kasl study, patients report feeling healthier than observers would say they are.

Above, we argued for the predictive validity of patients' own estimates of their health. Here, we wish to focus on the gaps in mutual understanding that such studies reveal, gaps that probably go unrecognized by everyone but the few researchers who tease them out. Patients typically interact with doctors, nurses, and loved ones with blithe confidence that they are understood, and these others undoubtedly feel they do understand. Where the discrepancies come from is unknown. Patients' needs for optimism or acceptance may lead them to deny their disabilities, as we suggested; alternatively, those who look out for them may have their own needs to see disability. Yet another possibility is that other people think a patient is doing worse than the patient thinks because the patient tends to communicate negative feelings and experiences more than positive ones. The question "how are you?" inevitably brings forth a list of problems that could, in turn, bias the questioner's overall understanding of the patient's state. But, regardless of the explanation, it is obvious that providers, family, and patients do not share a common understanding of the patient's experience of health and illness.

The famous dictum of the nineteenth-century physician Sir William Osler, "Listen to the patient, he is telling you the diagnosis" (Osler, 1904), is echoed by the conclusions of the Yale researchers, referred to earlier: "Knowledge that expressions of subjective health status are sensitive indications of survival length should engender new respect among health professionals for what people, especially the elderly people they treat, are saying about their health" (Idler & Kasl, 1991, p. 65).

BEYOND BIOMEDICINE TO THE PATIENT'S EXPERIENCE OF LIFE

This brings us to the third communication-transforming principle: *Communication should facilitate recognition of the link between a patient's mental state and the physical experience of illness.* Communication should go beyond biomedicine to reflect and respect the patient's experience of life.

Many—in fact, most—medical symptoms for which patients seek medical care cannot be tied to a specific diagnosis. The reason for this failure is that these are not symptoms of disease, in the medical sense, but are reactions to life. Headaches, rashes, dizziness, fatigue, stomach disorders, aches, chronic constipation or diarrhea, and weight fluctuations may very well reflect problems of living rather than underlying disease. People experience stress every day and in every circumstance—certainly everyone has suffered at some time over a stressful job, family relationships, or money. It is not uncommon for patients to express their distress in genuine physical symptoms such as those listed above. In fact, people experiencing life stresses are very high users of health services for physical complaints that are never linked to any organic problem, and, in fact, these patients take the lion's share of physicians' time.

What is most frustrating for patients experiencing physical symptoms related to life stresses is how difficult it is to communicate these problems to their physicians. Whereas patients may be describing their experiences from the perspective of their "lifeworld" (Mishler, 1984), physicians are interpreting symptoms from their technological perspective. A patient may feel discouraged from talking about "nonmedical" things such as stresses because this may not seem appropriate (or important enough) for the medical encounter, or because of a perception that the doctor can't do anything about it anyway.

Both patients and physicians need to know this is not the case. Through the talk of the medical visit, the doctor and patient can often find effective ways to address the physical manifestation, as well as the contributing underlying distress. Rather than an irritating distraction from the "business of medicine," problems with emotional and stress dimensions constitute a major component of medical practice.

As pointed out by K. L. White (1988) in his summary of the literature of medical efficacy, it is exactly these cases, these "distractions," that are the mainstay of medicine. K. L. White maintained that about a quarter of all benefits to be derived from medical care cannot be attributed to either technical expertise and agents or to the placebo or Hawthorne effect (that is, a positive response stemming from the sheer fact of being the object of attention). K. L. White attributed the therapeutic effect of talk to this unnamed and mysterious power.

PHYSICIANS AS EXPERTS

A singularly consistent finding in studies of doctors and patients conducted over the past 25 years has been that patients want as much information as possible from their physicians. Here is the fourth communication-enhancing principle: *Physicians have the duty to share their medical expertise with patients in such a way that this information is clear, relevant, and useful to patients.*

The first definition for "doctor" in Webster's dictionary is "teacher." The word "teacher" implies helping, but this help is not limited to the usual clinical sense of providing the correct diagnosis and treatment, or empathy and reassurance. A teacher helps by equipping learners (patients) with what they need to help themselves; this includes not only information, but also confidence in the value of their own contributions. The educator model is thus more egalitarian and collaborative than the traditional doctor-patient model, and, as such, is well suited to a literate and consumerist society such as ours. In contrast, Paulo Freire (1970), a well-known educator, described the traditional model of education in which teachers deposit knowledge and directives for living into passive recipients as though they were empty vessels or bank accounts; indeed, he called this the "banking" method of education. Freire advocated instead a relationship between teacher and learner that acknowledges what learners can impart to teachers.

Thus, his model is one in which learning goes both ways and the teacher-learner distinction is considerably blurred.

Applying this to the doctor-patient relationship, one can imagine greater mutual recognition of the unique store of knowledge possessed by the patient, which can be as crucial for a positive treatment outcome as the physician's biomedical knowledge is. The medical visit is truly a "meeting between experts" (Tuckett et al., 1985). Even if one prefers the more traditional concept of the doctor alone as the expert, the doctor still has responsibility to educate patients. Most doctors do recognize this, up to a point, but a critical difference between our conception of a true educator and the traditional doctor model is that the educator, by considering the patient's expertise, can share knowledge in a way that is most meaningful to the patient. Though we are not suggesting that physicians should try to share the most technical aspects of their knowledge with patients, it is in fact the case that the knowledge most pertinent to most patients' conditions is easily conveyed and readily understood. The imparting of this information creates a spirit of collegiality that enhances a patient's ability and willingness to make informed decisions and meaningful commitments to treatment.

A good case in point is the tremendous problem of patient noncompliance—failure to do what the doctor recommends. Studies of noncompliance report that 10 to 90% of patients do not fully follow their doctors' orders, with most researchers in agreement that at least half of all patients do not take their prescribed drugs correctly (DiMatteo, 2004). Adherence to diet, exercise, alcohol restrictions, and other lifestyle changes is probably far worse. The extent of noncompliance is much more widespread than most doctors estimate, and appreciation for the problems reflected by these terribly low figures is very often simplistic. For example, when dealing with patients whose high blood pressure remains uncontrolled, too often the focus is persistently on drugs; the task is to find the "right" one, the one with the proper biochemical composition. But a more fruitful search would be for a better understanding of the patient rather than the drug. Does the patient take the drugs as prescribed? What is the patient's perspective on high blood pressure? Is it viewed as a meaningless measurement associated with nonsymptoms that (illogically) lead to a need for drugs? Does the patient see no reason to continue to take the drug when he or she feels well? Does the patient stop if he or she feels worse? Are there side effects that interfere with valued social activities? Are the drugs too expensive?

Attention to these kinds of issues might lead not only to a more accurate assessment of the extent of noncompliance, but also to a negotiation between doctor and patient regarding the most appropriate treatment plan and tailored interventions that address social, behavioral, and emotional factors associated with compliance (Roter, Hall, Merisca, Ruehle, Cretin, &

Svarstad, 1998). The result would therefore be not only a concrete plan but a "customer approach to patienthood" that is much more likely to lead to compliance because the treatment plan makes sense to patients, is compatible with their lifestyles, and reflects their own input (Golin, DiMatteo, & Gelberg, 1996; Lazare, Eisenthal, & Wasserman, 1975). Moreover, the result is also likely to enhance patients' satisfaction with physicians. And, if patients like their physicians and trust not only their technical skill but also their commitment to advocate a plan of treatment that really is best suited for the patients, the patients are more likely to comply. The physician's negotiating behavior, the full and open exchange of ideas, is the ground from which springs the patient's motivation to comply.

THE COMMUNICATION OF EMOTIONS

Though patients certainly want information and services from their physicians, these are not the only things that patients want. Physicians are not simply expert consultants, although they are that; they are also someone to whom people go when they are particularly vulnerable and with whom they form bonds. This brings us to the fifth communication-transforming principle: *Communication carries emotional significance, and the expression, recognition, and response to emotion shape the nature of the relationship that is developed between a patient and his or her doctor.*

Considering that a large portion of medical care is based on interpersonal interaction—albeit a very special kind of interaction—all the processes that characterize interaction in general are applicable. In fact, all exchanges between doctors and patients carry cues about feelings and attitudes. People emit cues that are given meaning whether they want to or not. Thus, a distressed patient who tries to conceal his or her agitation may "leak" such cues anyway. A physician who equates professionalism with a neutral demeanor and emotional distance will most likely react in spontaneous expressive ways in spite of these intentions—for example, by revealing irritation with a particularly troublesome patient or distress at having to convey bad news. Because emotions (and related phenomena such as desires, moods, and feelings) can be revealed through nonverbal cues as well as talked about with words, nonverbal behavior is very important in the medical visit. Though nonverbal behavior has not been ignored in the context of the medical visit (Heath, 1986; J. A. Hall, Harrigan, & Rosenthal, 1995), it has clearly not received the attention it deserves.

There are three interrelated ways that emotions play a part in the process of medical care. First, both physicians and patients have emotions. Both physicians and patients are influenced by emotions they have experienced in the past, they experience emotions when interacting with each other, and they anticipate having emotions in the future. Emotions exert a profound influence on an individual's cognition and behavior, including prosocial acts, recollection, decision making, persuasion, information processing, and interpersonal attitudes (Oatley & Jenkins, 1996).

We often think of patients as the ones having emotions. For example, they may have anxiety or depression, and they are likely to have positive or negative feelings about their physicians. Physicians' emotions and their emotional responses to patients have received far less study than that of patients', although they are certainly present in equal measure. An antagonistic, frustrating, or demanding patient may anger or exasperate a physician (Levinson, 1993), while a pleasant, healthy, or cooperative patient may be liked more than others (J. A. Hall, Epstein, DeCiantis, & McNeil, 1993; J. A. Hall, Horgan, Stein, & Roter, 2002). A physician may be unaware of his or her emotional responses or may try to suppress them. Alternatively, a physician may try to orchestrate the visit so that emotionally demanding or arousing situations do not occur.

Second, both physicians and patients show emotions, sometimes in spite of efforts at suppression or masking. As examples, both physicians and patients reveal their liking of each other, at least enough so that they can each pick up on it at greater than chance levels (J. A. Hall et al., 2002). Some of the emotional cues that are conveyed by patients reflect their illness state. These include cues relating to physical pain (Prkachin, 1992; Patrick, Craig, & Prkachin, 1986) and to physical and psychological distress (J. A. Hall, Roter, Milburn, & Daltroy, 1996). Coronary disease is associated with distinctive vocal and facial expressions (Friedman, Hall, & Harris, 1985; J. A. Hall, Friedman, & Harris, 1986). Among patients with coronary illness, episodes of ischemia correspond with facial movements associated with anger, suggesting that anger can trigger coronary events (Rosenberg, et al., 2001). Some of the cues expressed by patients are inadvertently conveyed, while others are part of deliberate efforts to convey the experience of symptoms and suffering to the physician—experiences that are difficult to express in words (Heath, 2002).

Third, and finally, the evidence that emotions are shown in the medical visit implies that both physicians and patients judge each other's emotions. Patients do this to gain insight into how physicians feel about them, and physicians do this to gain insight into how patients feel about them. (This is illustrated by the accuracy with which physicians can judge how much they are liked by their patients and the accuracy with which patients can judge how much they are liked by their physicians.) The judgment of emotion may also be taken as a clue to hidden or obscured information reflecting an individual's inner state (both physical and emotional). Physicians use patients' affective cues in the diagnostic process, as well as in evaluating clinical progress and overall well-being. For example, physicians may elicit emotions to help make a diagnosis such as expressive aphasia, or may look for certain nonverbal cues when concerned about a patient's possible depression. Patients may also use physicians' affective cues in a sort of parallel diagnostic process to draw conclusions about the doctor, as well as about the veracity and seriousness of the information that is conveyed. Using information derived from both what the doctor says and how he or she says it, patients may judge the kind of person the doctor is and the nature of the doctor's attitudes, intentions, and trustworthiness. Thus, even a doctor who is bland in expression and who spends all his or her time on medical business may still inspire good feelings in a patient because the patient values being taken seriously. Further, physicians who provide adequate information are likely to be interpreted as being competent and caring, and these interpretations may be a major influence on the relationship and the entire course of illness; these interpretations may be more important even than the information itself.

Patients also look to physicians for "information behind the information" in an attempt to come to terms with the uncertainty and anxiety that so often accompanies health-threatening or life-threatening conditions. Is there yet more bad news to come? Is there reason to hope? Has the doctor given up on me? The judgments physicians and patients make of each other's emotional cues may be right or wrong, but, either way, such judgments are likely to lead to behavioral choices and possibly to health consequences.

RECIPROCITY

Negotiation and bargaining, reflecting the parties' concepts of fairness and deserving, are implicit in any relationship, including that of doctor and patient. The sixth communication-transforming principle is based on this notion of reciprocity: *Doctors and patients continually evaluate the adequacy of each other's performance, according to their own values and expectations, and respond in a way that they feel somehow matches with, or is deserved by, the other's behavior.*

The common notion of reciprocity centers on things people can do for, or give to, each other in a spirit of exchange. This exchange includes both feelings and calculations. In medical encounters, there seems to be a trade-off between good feelings and coolly calculated obligation. When feelings of gratitude, love, or esteem are strong, a sense of obligation is scarcely felt, and the desire to do something for another feels spontaneous: a deed is done because the person wants to. But when positive feelings are not so strong, a sense of obligation emerges, and reciprocity becomes a duty, a "should." Under these circumstances, awareness of calculation is likely to be high, and calculation of what is due can be exceedingly detailed. Reciprocation as we are defining it need not be literally in kind—an exact tit for tat—but can represent a broad array of calibrated responses aimed at establishing psychological equity or emotional satisfaction.

In the medical relationship, a special case exists with regard to reciprocity. The doctor can do things for the patient, but the patient can do things both for the doctor and for himself or herself. Interestingly, because patients can choose between doctor-directed responses and responses on their own behalf, patients can hurt themselves. As an example, consider the situation in which Dr. Smith fails to provide Mr. Brown with a preferred drug. Mr. Brown may then express disappointment by less than full compliance with the drug that was prescribed. "Getting even" with objectionable physician behaviors can even lead patients to drop out of care altogether. Thus, the need for emotional equity can, ironically, lead patients to behave in ways that are not good for their health. Of course, reciprocity may work the other way as well, producing a positive rather than a negative spiral. The doctor who is perceived as working especially hard may find that the patient not only expresses gratitude, but may follow the prescribed regimen with special conscientiousness.

Exchanges can be literal: payment of bills following services rendered is expected. But many patients go beyond the expected payment by providing their doctors with gifts, particularly at Christmas, on special occasions, and after a serious illness (Drew, Stoeckle, & Billings, 1983). Patients who feel they did not receive the kind of care they expected may withhold payment of bills, boycott further services, discourage friends from going to this doctor, or even file malpractice suits. The psychological experience of the reciprocity norm in the doctor-patient relationship takes the form of each deciding what form of response or behavior is justified and deserved under the circumstances. Thus, minor disappointments might result in partial withholding of payment but larger disappointments might result in more drastic action.

Although dramatic gestures like those mentioned earlier clearly illustrate the reciprocity rule, more subtle reactions, as well as moment-to-moment acts within the medical visit, can also be seen in this light. Thus, positive statements or facial expressions by the doctor are likely to produce the same behavior in the patient. If a warm greeting pleases the patient, the patient returns good feeling (warm behavior) to the doctor. If one party behaves in a reserved manner, chances are that the other will behave coolly too. Behaviors that are more task oriented in both doctor and patient can also show reciprocity; for example, more information giving by the doctor and greater expertise produce better understanding and better patient compliance. Although some of these benefits are fostered directly by the information, we think an equally important force is the motive to repay that is aroused by the patient's perception of good doctor performance. It is also likely that the reciprocation of task-oriented behaviors with other task-oriented behaviors is fostered when a positive emotional climate exists between the doctor and patient. In daily life, as well as in physician-patient encounters, individuals often lack insight into the important ways in which their own behaviors produce the behaviors that they observe in others. Often, those behaviors are attributed to the other without the realization that the other is simply returning the kind of behavior he or she received.

Reciprocity can also occur when the doctor's and patient's behaviors look quite different on the surface. For example, a patient may respond with liking (an emotional reaction) to a doctor who is highly competent (a technical skill). Such a reaction would be reciprocity if, as mentioned above, the patient interprets such a doctor to be showing his own positive feelings for the patient by being so conscientious. What does not happen much, we think, is the reverse—a patient responding with task-oriented behaviors to a doctor's friendly personal style. Just this point was made through an experiment by Willson and McNamara (1982) that showed that people viewing taped vignettes of doctor-patient interactions interpreted a competent doctor to be courteous, but did not interpret a courteous one to be competent unless actual competence was portrayed. Courtesy and friendliness were not enough to convince patients of the doctor's expertise nor sufficient to guarantee commitment to the recommended regimen. Thus, patients are constantly making inferences about doctors, and doctors would do well to consider the impact of what they do and say on their patients.

Patients, for their part, need to be persuaded, perhaps even more than their doctors do, that they are important influencers too. Patients are more likely to feel like objects than like agents. However, doctors are profoundly influenced by the demeanor, interest, expressions, comments, attitudes, and positive or negative regard expressed by their patients. That influence can return to help or to haunt the patient. To take an extreme case, a patient who is consistently rude and irritable will almost certainly not receive the same medical care as a patient who conveys positive, or at least constructive, attitudes. More subtly, patients' expectations for how their physicians are going to act will very likely come true because the expectations shape the patient's behavior, which, by reciprocity, is reflected back in the behavior of the doctor.

CONFORMING TO NOTIONS OF "GOOD" DOCTOR AND "GOOD" PATIENT

Just as doctors and patients influence each other, each of them is also influenced by prior experiences, and these impact the medical visit. This brings us to the seventh communication-transforming principle: *Becoming more aware of roles and the assumptions and expectations they bring with them can help both participants gain a sense of power and the freedom to change within the medical encounter.* Well-learned roles such as those of doctor and patient are hard to change. One reason lies in the mostly unconscious manner in which people act out roles. Like speaking a well-rehearsed part or driving a car, the many words and actions that make up "acting like a doctor" and "acting like a patient" become automatic and are beyond conscious awareness.

One reason why people conform to the roles they are cast in is the practically mortal fear of committing social improprieties. This is especially pertinent to the patient role, which traditionally has been a rather passive one. We believe it is often a dread of being inappropriate, of doing the "wrong" thing, that prevents patients from offering their opinions, asking questions, or asking their doctors to show them their medical charts, even when such actions are clearly in the patients' best interest. Patients feel they are not supposed to do these things.

A different, but nonetheless limiting, attitude that patients often have is that the situation itself is a given—a "that's how it is" approach in which patients can do little more than fit into a system that is much more powerful than they are. Attendant on this passivity is the fear that failure to fit in will get one branded as a troublemaker or a crank. Extreme deviance would certainly produce bad effects in any social situation where norms are well established. But patients have more latitude than they think. As they prefer, they can ask more questions, demand more information, take control of certain decisions, read their charts, and in general use fully the time that they are paying for. Especially for patients, becoming more aware of roles can help liberate them from feeling they "have to" act certain ways. Roles, after all, are just a kind of conformity, not a moral code or rule of law.

For their part, doctors learn their role from their own observation of doctors they have had and from media portrayals and cultural values, but, most of all, the doctor role is learned in medical school. Medical education is designed not only to teach biochemistry and physiology but also to teach how one acts as a doctor. Unfortunately, the current training process is often dehumanizing; interns are forced to give up any semblance of a normal home life and typically work every other night at the hospital (Klass, 1987). This cannot help but create a callous view of patients: patients are but one more obstacle to seeing their families or getting some sleep. Even after training, many doctors feel their lives are unreasonably burdened by the stress of on-call responsibilities and hospital pressures, and these experiences can carry over into the medical visit in negative ways (Hilfiker, 1985).

Medical education could help young doctors to overcome this negative experience. As we see it, medical education can have two kinds of impact on doctor-patient relations. First, it can affect skills. Schools can teach doctors to do a variety of things better—to be better communicators and patient educators, to motivate patients more effectively, and to reassure and comfort them better. Second, it can help them think holistically about the kind of doctor they want to be. Critics of medical education have often argued that the emphasis on basic science is out of proportion to its relevance to clinical practice, and that interpersonal and communication skills, which are so critical, get short shrift in the medical curriculum. Indeed, in their early years of medical school, students do a better job of talking with their patients than fully trained doctors. A well-known study of medical education found that medical students' interpersonal skills with patients declined as their medical education progressed (Helfer, 1970). This was particularly true for the students' ability to take a good social history. It seems that, as students learned more about the "science" of medicine, they found it harder simply to talk with patients, and came to devalue this kind of activity. What were easy exchanges during the first years later became an awkward and unproductive series of closed-ended, usually yes-or-no, questions. No doubt related to this narrowing of focus, Martin et al. (1976) found that, as training progressed, physicians seemed increasingly to lose their grasp on the patient's total health picture and to focus more and more on biomedical issues.

Although the improvement of physicians' skills in interviewing is valuable, skill does not go to the heart of the matter. Medical school needs to do a better job of inculcating different attitudes in young doctors—in defining for them what is truly important about being a doctor and what are effective, and humane, doctor-patient roles. Our society must figure out how to influence their attitudes so that they come to value certain aspects of patient care differently. Then, of course, when these doctors become mentors themselves, they will provide a different kind of example to their students. If physicians saw themselves more as educators, we also believe medical education would be different, and the profession would engage in a different kind of self-scrutiny. More attention would be paid to the process of teaching, which would translate into a more sensitive involvement of doctors in the process of healing.

RECOGNITION OF RELATIONSHIP-CENTERED MEDICAL CARE

Taken as a whole, these seven principles provide a blueprint for the communication field. They represent the challenges and the potential for a transformation in medicine, not only in talk but also in the clinical model that underlies the practice of medicine. At their heart, the principles we describe reflect a single notion—that the process of care brings people

2

The Nature of the
Doctor-Patient Relationship

Once the patient and physician are brought together, they enter a relationship predicated on the expectations each holds for the conduct of the other. The relationship thus formed has substantial implications for how the curing and caring process will be accomplished and the extent to which needs and expectations will be met, satisfaction achieved, and health restored.

Critical to expectations regarding the conduct of the medical visit are varying perspectives on notions of authority and autonomy. Medical authority is viewed as part and parcel of the services of an expert—a patient follows the doctor's orders because it is assumed that the orders are scientifically based and well-meaning (Parsons, 1951, 1975). The physician's authority to direct patient behavior is conceded, and thus legitimated, by patients in light of the physician's advanced training and expertise. On occasion, however, patients may resist a doctor's orders and declare an intention to follow their own inclinations instead. This withdrawal of authority can be seen as an expression of patient autonomy—the power to resist the physician's will (Haug & Lavin, 1983).

There are two views regarding the potential clash between patient autonomy and physician authority in the doctor-patient relationship. The first is a consensual accommodation, and the second is outright conflict. The consensual view has been articulated by Talcott Parsons (1951, 1975), who argued that conflict is managed and diffused by well-defined societal expectations for both patient and physician conduct. In contrast, Freidson (1970) saw conflict as ongoing and fundamental to the doctor-patient relationship.

The most fully discussed area of conflict related to the autonomy/authority clash is the area of medical knowledge. In some respects, the argument over knowledge may be reduced to a question of ownership.

Parsons argued that, inherent in the definition of a physician, is the dedication of a lifetime to the mastery of knowledge and the gaining of experience in the application of that knowledge. The fund of medical knowledge is so vast and complex, the schooling so intense and grueling, and the daily experience so unique, that an unbridgeable competence gap exists between physicians and the lay world. Medical knowledge is thus earned and owned by doctors. Moreover, this knowledge is impossible to share. Because patients must accept medical practice on faith, they are afforded certain protections. Central to this protection is the higher code of moral conduct that physicians are held to, including a code of ethics defining the special duty of physicians to protect the interests of their patients. Patients, for their part, rely on physician adherence to this moral code and therefore cooperate with doctor's orders. Any conflict between doctor and patient is resolved by physician authority and the assumption that "the doctor knows best." A patient who resists doctor's orders risks potential loss of standing as a patient and the stigma of a malingerer or a fake; no patient can truly want to get well if he or she does not cooperate with the doctor.

A different view regarding the conflict over medical knowledge between physician authority and patient autonomy can be articulated. Though agreeing with Parsons that the predominant characteristic of the physician is the mastery of expert knowledge and experience, Freidson saw the disinclination of physicians to share information with patients less as a function of a competence gap than as a safeguard for high status and professional standing (Freidson, 1970). Moreover, a less knowledgeable patient is less likely to second-guess the doctor or detect medical errors.

In any given situation, a patient may fear that the physician has overlooked or denigrated a significant and important symptom because the physician's knowledge is flawed or incomplete. This may either be because of deficiencies in medical science or because of the personal failings of the physician (Freidson, 1960). The physician-to-patient ratio generally means that the physician cannot always give sufficient attention or time to any one patient or medical problem. Even if the physician fails only once in 10,000 cases, that is sufficient cause for an individual patient to wonder if he or she will be that case (Freidson, 1960). A share in the information base can assure a patient that this is not the case. Moreover, most patients highly value information as a way of coping with the uncertainty of illness and as a mechanism for greater participation in medical decision making. (The value and importance of information to patients is presented in further detail in Chapter 8.)

Professional knowledge, per se, is not all that is gained during medical training. Physicians also learn and internalize a worldview that includes a way of thinking based on the biomedical model of disease (Engel, 1977). The predominant view a physician brings to medical practice is one anchored in the world of biochemistry and technology. In contrast, a patient's world is comprised of a complex web of personality, culture, living situations, and relationships that color and define the illness experience (Kleinman, 1987; Mishler, 1984). The conflict is between incomplete perspectives: the biomedical view loses the context of the patient's life, while the patient's experience may lack insight into science and potential medical intervention.

A contest of definitions ensues between doctor and patient. The physician wants a biomedical definition, posed as a disease with known physical manifestations, which implies medical ownership, while the patient wants the definition to be his or her own in terms of his or her illness experience (Cassell, 1976; Mishler, 1984). The physician who dismisses a debilitating flu as "only the flu" may miss, from the patient's perspective, the full impact of the illness experience and its meaning. For the patient, the flu may be seen as an indication of a compromised immune system and an early sign of cancer. Failure to appreciate this kind of significance arises from a fundamental difference between doctors and patients in their worldview.

It is through manipulation of information and definition of the problem that the nature and conduct of the visit are determined—what will be said and done, when, and how. Patients have some measure of power over how the medical visit will proceed, although its expression is usually more subtle than the expression of the physician's power. Patients can withhold information from the physician—not giving a truthful or complete report of their medical condition, for instance—to create an impression of being more or less sick than they actually are (Roth, 1963). They can, of course, request and insist on certain procedures or prescriptions, ask questions and probe the physician's clinical reasoning, or refuse to go along with a recommended test or treatment. Direct confrontation between doctor and patient, however, is the exception rather than the rule. Far more common are maneuvers and negotiations that span a broad spectrum of power relations.

It is along this negotiated spectrum that patient autonomy and physician authority are defined in any given relationship. Because of the great variability in patients' ability to negotiate in this realm, ethicists have identified the potential for medical coercion as a central question of medical ethics. Indeed, since the 1960s, patient autonomy has become a tenet of medical ethics, and it is almost universally regarded as a necessary and important element of civilized and enlightened medical care (President's Commission for the Study of Ethical Problems in Medicine and Biomedical and Behavioral Research, 1982).

Table 2.1
Types of Doctor-Patient Relationships

Patient Control	Physician Control	
	Low	High
Low	Default	Paternalism
High	Consumerism	Mutuality

To further explore the varying perspectives on the doctor-patient relationship, four alternative ideal models of this relationship will be discussed.

PROTOTYPES OF CONTROL IN THE DOCTOR-PATIENT RELATIONSHIP

Bioethicists E. J. Emanuel and L. L. Emanuel (1992) suggest that power relations in medical visits are expressed through several key elements, including (1) who sets the agenda and goals of the visit (the physician, the physician and patient in negotiation, or the patient); (2) the role of the patient's values (assumed by the physician to be consistent with his or her own, jointly explored by the patient and the physician, or unexamined); and (3) the functional role assumed by the physician (guardian, advisor, or consultant). The expression of power, and the dynamics of negotiation, can take several forms, each shaping a markedly different relationship. Table 2.1 illustrates the four ideal forms of the doctor-patient relationship: paternalism, consumerism, mutuality, and default.

Most prevalent, but not necessarily the most efficient or desirable, the prototype of *paternalism* is shown in the upper-right quadrant of Table 2.1. In this model of relations, physicians dominate agenda setting, goal setting, and decision making with regard to both information and services; the medical condition is defined in biomedical terms, and the patient's voice is largely absent. The physician's obligation is to act in the patient's "best interest." The determination of best interest, however, is largely based on the assumption that the patient's values and preferences are the same as those of the physician. The guiding model is that of the physician as the guardian, acting in the patient's best interest regardless of the patient's preferences. The patient's job is to cooperate with medical advice, that is, to do what he or she is told.

The lower-left quadrant of Table 2.1 represents *consumerism*. Here the more typical power relationship between doctors and patients may be reversed. Patients set the goals and agenda of the visit and take sole responsibility for decision making. The patient's demands for information and technical services are accommodated by a cooperating physician. The patient's values are defined and fixed by the patient and are unexamined by the physician. This type of relationship redefines the medical encounter as a marketplace transaction. Caveat emptor, "let the buyer beware," rules the transaction, with power resting in the buyer (patient) who can make the decision to buy (seek care) or not, as the patient sees fit (Haug & Lavin, 1983). The physician's role is limited to that of a technical consultant who has the obligation to provide information and services that are contingent on the patient's preferences (and within professional norms).

While still stressing patient control, the prototype of *mutuality,* shown in the lower-right quadrant of Table 2.1 proposes a more moderate alternative to the extremes of paternalism and consumerism. In this model, each participant brings strengths and resources to the relationship on a relatively even footing. Inasmuch as power in the relationship is balanced, the goals, agenda, and decisions related to the visit are the result of negotiation between partners; both the patient and the physician become part of a joint venture. Medical dialogue is the vehicle through which the patient's values are explicitly articulated and explored. Throughout this process, the physician acts as a counselor or advisor.

It is also within the mutuality model that the concept of the relationship itself is elevated to a new status. Although all of the models suppose the doctor-patient relationship to be the context within which the different roles exist, the concept of "being in a relationship" has intrinsic value for both the doctor and the patient. The emphasis shifts from the acting of complementary roles to the expression of mutual personhood. In this model, dialogue and the mutual expression of feelings are seen as holding great therapeutic potential (Beach & Inui, 2006).

What happens when the patient's and the physician's expectations are at odds or when the need for change in the relationship cannot be negotiated? A possible consequence of a poor "fit," or the failure to change the relationship as needs and circumstances change, is a relationship *default,* which is represented in the upper-left quadrant of Table 2.1 and is characterized by a lack of control by either the patient or the physician. It is in this case that a patient may drop out of care completely because of failed expectations or frustrated goals.

Contrasting perspectives from the research literature have been drawn to illustrate each of the four models of the doctor-patient relationship.

PATERNALISM

Paternalism is widely regarded as the traditional form of the doctor-patient relationship, and it is still seen as the most common one (E. J. Emanuel & L. L. Emanuel, 1992; President's Commission for the Study of Ethical Problems in Medicine and Biomedical and Behavioral Research,

1982; Szasz & Hollender, 1956). A passive patient and a dominant physician as the idealized therapeutic relationship is most clearly articulated by Parsons in his classic writings on the role of the sick (Parsons, 1951). Parsons saw the doctor and patient as fulfilling necessary functions in a well-balanced and maintained social structure. Sickness, in this model, is considered to be a necessary, occasional respite, providing a brief exemption for patients from societal responsibilities. However, for society to continue to function, this respite must be controlled. By defining the terms of the illness and its privileges, physicians provide this controlling force.

When sick, a patient is allowed the privileges of convalescence—he or she is not held responsible for poor health and is excused from everyday responsibilities. However, in order to enjoy these privileges, the patient must seek technically competent help and comply with medical advice. The patient's role is thus passive and dependent. In contrast, the doctor's role is defined as professionally dominant and autonomous. The doctor legitimates the patient's illness and determines the course of treatment. In doing so, the physician is compelled by professional ethics to act only in his or her sphere of expertise, to maintain an emotional detachment and distance from the patient, and to act in the patient's best interest.

From a societal perspective, this model is argued to be more functional than others. The authority afforded physicians provides the weight necessary for the important certification role of physicians in determining how sick a patient is and how much leeway will be given to him or her. This might include leeway in terms of exemptions from work and home responsibilities, as well as economic compensation for disabilities associated with work-related accidents. Moreover, it is the physicians' authority that gives them their ability to reintegrate patients back into society at the end of their sickness episodes. The physician is the one who determines when health is restored and when sick privileges should be withdrawn.

In addition to the social control function that the paternalism model offers, there are significant nurturing and supportive aspects to this type of relationship. Patients may draw comfort and support from a doctor ("father") figure. Indeed, the supportive nature of paternalism appears to be all the more important when patients are very sick and at their most vulnerable (Ende, Kazis, Ash, & Moskowitz, 1989; Ende, Kazis, & Moskowitz, 1990). Relief from the burden of worry is curative in itself, some argue, and the trust and confidence implied by this model allow the doctor to perform "medical magic." There is also evidence that idealization of the physician can have an important therapeutic effect, as placebo studies have demonstrated (Lasagna, Mosteller, von Feisinger, & Beecher, 1954).

What, then, is the problem? How is it that medical paternalism has become identified as a particular danger from which patients need to be protected? It is the potential for legitimate medical authority to be used for manipulation and exploitation of the vulnerable and ill that has fueled the ascendance of the autonomy doctrine to the preeminent bioethical value in patient-physician relationships (Schneider, 1998). That protections against medical authority have been widespread is reflected in the colorful comments of bioethicist Arthur Caplan: "The Freddy Kruger of bioethics for the better part of two decades has been the doctor who pushes his or her values onto the patient. . . . This devil has been completely exorcised and a large part of contemporary bioethics scholarship seems to be devoted to the task of assuring that the paternalistic doctor stays dead and buried" (Caplan, as cited in Schneider, 1998, p. 4). The victory over medical paternalism, however, may only be illusory. More often than is openly acknowledged by the law or bioethicists, the procedures established to assure patient autonomy in informed consent and treatment decision making have become pro forma and useless autonomy rituals (Schneider, 1998).

The autonomy principle, Schneider (1998) argues, has been transformed from a doctrine that entitles, but does not require, the patient to take an active role in treatment decision making, to a view that treats patients as morally obligated to act autonomously. The doctrine of patient autonomy has gone beyond a principle of medical conduct, that is, from prescribing how doctors should treat patients to prescribing how patients should conduct themselves. Not only have patients lost the right to decide not to decide, but to decline to assume the obligations and responsibilities of mandatory autonomy is viewed as a moral failing that is deserving of contempt and blame. The objectives of the autonomy paradigm are often pursued regardless of the patient's preference for, reluctance toward, or incompetence when assuming an autonomous role in the medical relationship. Indeed, there are some patients, and perhaps many patients at especially vulnerable junctures and in particular circumstances, who do not want to or who cannot assume the burden for their medical decisions.

Relatively little is known about what kinds of patients are likely to prefer more paternalistic relationships with their physicians. Several sociodemographic variables do appear to be associated with this relationship preference. The strongest of these is older age, but lower income and lower level of occupation are also associated with this preference (Ende et al., 1989; Haug & Lavin, 1983; Pendleton & House, 1984). Other investigators have suggested that it is the wide gap in educational background and socioeconomic status between most patients and their physicians that contributes to the deference of lower–social class patients and their adoption of a passive and dependent role in the doctor-patient relationship (Pratt, Seligmann, & Reader, 1957; Waitzkin, 1985). Also citing the disparity in status and education between patients and physicians, the President's

Commission for the Study of Ethical Problems in Medicine and Biomedical and Behavioral Research (1982) concluded that, even when patients
and physicians have mutually agreed upon a paternalistic relationship,
questions regarding its appropriateness may still be raised. The Commission argued that patients and doctors are often on so unequal a footing that
few patients can really play an equal role with physicians in shaping the
relationship. The possibility exists, then, that patients may adopt a passive
patient role, because they are not fully aware of their alternatives or able
to negotiate a more active stance.

A difficulty in much of the literature, and in the work cited above, is
the wide range of definitions used to define the passive patient role. Several investigators (Strull, Lo, & Charles, 1984; Vertinsky, Thompson, &
Uyeno, 1974) have defined the active patient role as including the
decision-making prerogative in the therapeutic relationship, and, by
extension, a passive patient role as the patient's deference to the physician
in decision-making situations. A now well-replicated finding, using this
definition, is that patients show rather weak interest in assuming the
responsibility for medical decision making (Ende et al., 1989; Ende et al.,
1990; Pendleton & House, 1984; Strull et al., 1984; Vertinsky et al.,
1974). While a patient's decision-making preference has shown a weak
association with sociodemographic and knowledge variables, far stronger relationships have been found with illness severity (Ende et al.,
1989; Ende et al., 1990). This suggests that it is being ill that determines
a patient's decision-making preference, rather than the patient's knowledge and social status, as argued earlier. If illness severity is the critical
variable, as Ende and colleagues hypothesized, then physicians themselves, when they are under the care of a doctor, would relinquish their
autonomy in the same way as other patients. In studying such a situation,
Ende and colleagues (Ende et al., 1989; Ende et al., 1990) surveyed 151
physicians and 315 patients, attending a university medical clinic, on their
decision-making preferences. There was a significant but small difference
in decision-making preference between the physicians and the patients,
with physicians having a slightly higher preference for decision making
than patients (41 versus 34 on a 100-point scale), but their preference was
still short of favoring equal participation.

Findings from the study suggested that physicians, like the regular
patients in the study, preferred that the principal role in decision making for
their illnesses be taken by the doctor, not by themselves (Ende et al., 1990).
Moreover, as the severity of the illness increased, the tendency of
physician-patients was to rely even more on their own physicians for decision making. Because the physicians in this study responded so similarly to
the patients, the investigators concluded that medical knowledge and socio-

cultural factors are only minor determinants of patients' attitudes towards autonomy, while illness severity appears to play a more critical role.

CONSUMERISM

The advent of medical consumerism in this country has been attributed to several significant societal changes since the 1960s (Reeder, 1972). The first of these is the shift from curative to preventive services. Reeder noted that, in a system dominated by curative or emergency care, there is a "seller's market," and the relationship tends to be characterized by the patient as the supplicant. However, when prevention of illness is emphasized, the patient is less a supplicant than a skeptic. Part of the doctor's job is to convince the patient of the necessity of noncurative services such as periodic checkups. Under these circumstances, there are elements of a "buyer's market" and a tendency for the "customer to be right."

Another feature of societal change, described by Reeder, is the development of consumerism as a social movement and the redefinition of a person as a consumer rather than a patient. In a similar vein, a concurrent critical focus on the bureaucratization of the system of medical care delivery and its spiraling costs has resulted in an increasing use of the term "health care provider" to replace the more traditional terms "doctor" and "physician." Redefinition of the doctor-patient relationship as a consumer-provider exchange is more than a matter of simple semantics, for it refocuses the traditional perspective and thereby changes the very nature of the social relationship between the medical profession and the lay world (Reeder, 1972). Several authors have defined consumerism as the patients' challenge to unilateral decision making by physicians in reaching closure on diagnoses and working out treatment plans (Haug & Lavin, 1983). Inherent in this definition is a challenge to physician authority by reversing the very basic nature of the power relationship:

> [I]t focuses on the purchaser's (patient's) rights and seller's (physician's) obligations, rather than on physician's rights (to direct) and patient obligations (to follow directions). . . . In a consumer relationship, the seller has no particular authority; if anything, legitimated power rests in the buyer, who can make the decision to buy or not to buy, as he or she sees fit. (Haug & Lavin, 1981, p. 213)

Because of the marketplace emphasis on consumerism, and societal concern with medical costs, it is not surprising that some investigators have focused consumerist behavior on cost-related issues. An emphasis on the economic ramifications of consumerism has stressed the consumer's role in making cost-conscious choices among insurance options and providers, using services more sparingly, and being more selective in the acceptance of provider advice, based on its cost (Hibbard & Weeks, 1987).

An illustrative study of the consumer as a cost-conscious health shopper was conducted by Hibbard and Weeks (1985). These investigators interviewed almost 2,000 consumers (half were working-age government employees, and half were Medicare enrollees who were over 65 years of age) to determine the extent to which they behaved in a consumerist manner. Indications of consumerism were (1) cost-consciousness—considering the physician's fees when selecting a physician, choosing not to see a physician when ill because of the cost, or asking about fees in discussions with a physician; (2) information seeking—reading health columns or articles or using health or medical reference books; (3) exercising independent judgment—following the doctor's instructions precisely or using one's own judgment in following the doctor's orders; and (4) consumer knowledge—responding knowledgeably to a six-question test of consumer sophistication.

The investigators reported that a minority of respondents engaged in consumer-like behaviors, with 39% of the respondents being classified as cost-sensitive, 37% as health information seekers, and 34% as using independent judgment in following a doctor's advice. Moreover, the Medicare population scored substantially lower on all of these indicators than did the working-age population. Overall, the results indicated that those with greater education, as well as those in younger age groups, were most likely to engage in consumerist behaviors. Respondents who reported having greater faith in doctors, and being more dependent on them, were much less likely than others to adopt a consumerist orientation.

Older respondents appeared especially unwilling to act independent of medical authority and exercise independent judgment. The authors suggested that the older respondents may have a different perception of the expected and proper role of the patient in health care. An exception to the elderly's deference to physicians, however, was evident among those who had greater experience with the health care system and for whom economic issues held greater salience. Out-of-pocket costs and the perception of health care costs as a burden were not only associated with cost consciousness, but also with information seeking, exercising independent judgment, and consumer knowledge—even among older Medicaid respondents. In a somewhat similar vein, an earlier study by these investigators also found that individuals over the age of 55, particularly females who were well-educated and generally skeptical of the medical profession, were more likely to obtain a physician fee guide than other people (Hibbard & Weeks, 1985).

The finding that faith in, and dependency on, physicians was an important barrier to the adoption of a consumerist orientation led the authors to conclude that patients need help not just in learning about cost issues but in making the transition from the traditional passive patient to a consumer. This would include stressing less common components of consumerism, such as when to seek care, how to negotiate successfully in the medical encounter, whether to accept medical advice, and where to seek alternative sources of information (Hibbard & Weeks, 1987).

An exploration of the extent to which patients were actually adopting a consumerist approach in medical visits, and the nature of physicians' responses to such a challenge, was undertaken by Haug and Lavin (1983). Based on a survey of 466 laypeople and 86 physicians, the investigators found that substantial percentages of both the public and physicians (60% and 81%, respectively) espoused attitudes consistent with a consumerist perspective. However, the extent of commitment to a consumerist model dropped when actual behavior was assessed. About half the public reported actual instances of challenging behavior, with 30% reporting a single instance of confrontation and 17% reporting two or more.

Survey respondents who were more rejecting of authority in general, more skeptical of physicians' service orientation, younger, and better educated were more likely to express consumerist attitudes. Reports of consumerist behaviors, however, were more likely to come from those who questioned physician competence, believed medical error occurred in their care, and were younger.

The view from physicians was different. Despite the high level of endorsement of consumerist attitudes, only 8% of physicians indicated that they had accommodated patients' demands for decision-making power. Approximately half the physicians indicated that they used persuasion, when challenged, to convince a patient of the appropriateness of their recommendation rather than, as the other half did, relying on traditional authority. The physicians who were more likely to accommodate patient's requests expressed more "modern" attitudes, including the denigration of authority in general and a belief in the fallibility of the physician. As one might expect, these physicians also held positive views of patients who raise questions.

When things seem to go wrong, when satisfaction is low, or when a patient suspects less than optimal care or outcome, patients are more likely to question physician authority (Ende et al., 1989; Haug & Lavin, 1983; Vertinsky et al., 1974) and to adopt a more active role in the doctor-patient relationship. As is evident from the work described earlier, patients' requests may be negotiated and accommodated or they may be perceived as confrontational and critical.

When medical or service requests by the patient are within the boundaries of good medical judgment (and, for most conditions, these boundaries are set quite wide), accommodation can occur with little conflict emerging. When these demands are contrary to standard practice, however, the physician is skirting the mainstream of medicine and risking ostracism and ridicule by medical colleagues. The reluctance to share decision-making responsibility with patients may be established early on during medical training, when heavy stress is put on physician control in order to carry out medical responsibilities, even if this is over patient objections (Haug & Lavin, 1983).

An example of a physician's accommodation of a patient's requests is provided by Norman Cousins's account of his recovery from a rare, life-threatening disease. Cousins relates how, while hospitalized, he presented his physician with his decision to try extremely high doses of vitamin C to treat his disease. He also decided to stop taking all other medications. Cousins's statement about his doctor is quite telling:

> I was incredibly fortunate to have as my doctor a man who knew that his biggest job was to encourage to the fullest the patient's will to live and to mobilize all the natural resources of body and mind to combat disease. Dr. Hitzig was willing to set aside the large and often hazardous armamentarium of powerful drugs . . . when he became convinced that his patient might have something better to offer. (Cousins, 1979, p. 44)

According to Cousins, his doctor agreed to the course of treatment because he really could offer no alternatives and because he knew that he could best serve his patient by encouraging the will to live and the need to feel some control over so overwhelming an illness.

While this case of physician accommodation may seem unusual, in fact there is little evidence that the more traditional course of treatment in this instance would have been more effective. As noted by Brody (1980), medicine is not an accomplished science. There are tremendous gaps in knowledge. Indeed, it has been estimated that the effectiveness of treatments is unknown for about 90% of the medical conditions seen in routine practice (Pickering, 1979). Moreover, many medical decisions are as related to the physician's personality and social characteristics as they are to the nature of the medical problem itself (Eisenberg, 1979).

MUTUALITY

Just as the paternalistic model can be criticized for its "physician-centric" exclusion of the patient's perspective, fault can also be found with the consumerist model as being too narrowly "patient-centric" by restricting the physician's role to that of technical consultant and thereby limiting the benefit that can be derived from the inclusion of the physician's perspective in the care process. The optimal doctor-patient relationship model, then, may be one that mutually embraces the contributions of both. The mutuality model views neither the patient nor the physician as standing alone, or as standing aside, when the difficult task of medical decision making is undertaken. Each of the participants brings strengths and resources to the relationship, as well as a commitment to work through disagreements in a mutually respectful manner.

Some 25 years ago, Brody (1980) identified four steps by which the physician can encourage mutuality. These include (1) the establishment of an atmosphere conducive to participation, which is achieved by enhancing the patient's perception that his or her contributions are appropriate and appreciated; (2) the ascertainment of the patient's goals and expectations; (3) the education of the patient about the nature of his or her problem, including a discussion of the pros and cons of alternative evaluation and treatment approaches, and a presentation and explanation of the physician's recommendations; and (4) the elicitation of the patient's informed suggestions and preferences and the negotiation of any disagreements between physician and patient.

In a more concrete formalization of mutuality, Quill (1983) has suggested the adoption of contract language to make the nature of patient and physician rights and responsibilities explicit. The starting point of the contract is the delineation of the patient's problem(s) and requested intervention(s). This is a two-way process; the patient needs to define his or her problem in an open and full manner, and the physician needs to work with the patient to articulate the problem and refine the request. Once expectations are verbalized, a process of negotiation can begin. Some requests can be filled with little difficulty; some requests need only minor modifications; some requests require a good deal of compromise, discussion, and debate; and, finally, some requests must be denied because they are patently harmful or violate the physician's sense of ethics and good judgment. Stressing the consensual, rather than the obligatory, nature of the relationship, Quill emphasizes the patient's right to seek care elsewhere when demands are not satisfactorily met, and the physician's right to withdraw services formally from a patient if he or she feels it is impossible to satisfy the patient's demands or achieve the treatment objectives.

Other authors have suggested that a very different kind of process, one in which physicians assist patients in stating their values regarding particular decisions, is the most desirable method by which a mutual, collaborative exchange may take place (Speedling & Rose, 1985). Deciding on a course of treatment for breast cancer, for example, which might include a radical mastectomy as opposed to a more limited surgery augmented by radiation and chemotherapy, is a decision that can be best made by explicitly working through its implications for a woman's self-image, her tolerance for side effects, and her issues of sexuality. On a less formal level, this same goal may be achieved by linking a general exploration of values related to health, sexuality, independence, and even dying, to meaningfully elucidate the dimensions of decision making with regard to treatment options.

One might question whether any physician, even a communication expert, could or would really take the time to explore a patient's values. This question was addressed in a descriptive study of the best and normative practices in end-of-life discussions (Roter, Larson, Fischer, Arnold, & Tulsky, 2000). Audiotape recordings of 56 visits conducted by physicians, identified through reputation or publication as experts in the fields of bioethics or communication, and 48 visits conducted by primary care physicians that included advanced directives discussions were compared. The audiotapes revealed that expert physicians practiced a different kind of medicine than other physicians, at least in regard to end-of-life discussions; experts spent more time on these discussions, were more likely to probe and elicit patients' values and experiences related to end-of-life issues, provided more resources and encouragement to their patients for decision making, and more effectively concluded the discussion, assuring that it ended with mutual understanding and no lingering questions or concerns. Inasmuch as the experts in this study truly practice what they preach, we can have some confidence, not only that the exploration of patient values is possible, but that training and mentoring by experts may indeed make these skills commonplace in the future.

Engagement in this process may be seen as fulfilling the provider's responsibility by assuring that medical expertise is fully utilized. The prospect of making an important therapeutic decision without guidance and support can be overwhelming to a patient. Decision making cannot be expected to take place within a therapeutic vacuum; real communication is not simply the communication of a treatment catalog. Meaningful exchange is the give-and-take necessary for an understanding of the patient's perspective by the provider and an appreciation for the options and their consequences, in terms of daily life, by the patient.

Beyond these conceptualizations of mutuality, the term "relationship-centered care" was coined in the early 1990s by the Pew-Fetzer Task Force on Advancing Psychosocial Health Education to recognize the therapeutic power of the doctor-patient relationship itself as more than simply the meeting of patient and physician for the performance of a technically appropriate transaction (Tresolini, 1994). As later elaborated by the Relationship-Centered Care Research Network (Beach & Inui, 2006), relationship-centered care differs from earlier models of mutuality and patient-centeredness because it emphasizes the dimension of personhood, that of both the patient and the physician; it also emphasizes how the expression, recognition, and reciprocation of emotion mutually influence the doctor and patient in relationship with one another and in relationship with the broader medical care community. In this model, dialogue is seen as the vehicle for the development of the doctor-patient relationship, which has, in itself, therapeutic potential. The concept of "being in a relationship" is itself a value to strive for, for both the doctor and the patient (Beach & Inui, 2006).

DEFAULT

When patient and physician expectations are at odds, or when the need for change in the relationship cannot be negotiated, the relationship may come to a dysfunctional standstill, a kind of relationship default. Default can be characterized by unclear or contested common goals and an uncertain physician role. It is here where medical management may be least effective, with neither the patient nor the physician sensing progress or direction. A frustrated and angry patient may make inappropriate time and service demands and may ultimately drop out of care completely because of failed expectations. For physicians, these visits represent the most frustrating aspects of medicine, reflecting "the difficult and hateful patient." Unless recalibration of the relationship is undertaken with direct intervention, the relationship is likely to continue to unravel and ultimately fail (Levinson, 1993).

A poorly functioning relationship may continue for a long time, without direction, or may terminate without any resolution. It is in this case that a patient may drop out of care completely because of failed expectations or frustrated goals, reflecting bitterly on the unresponsiveness of doctors. The physician might be unaware of the reasons for the loss of this patient. Indeed, the physician may not even realize that this patient has dropped out of care, as the patient will simply not come back. In the worst of scenarios, when a medical outcome has gone bad, the physician may become aware of a failed relationship through a malpractice complaint. Although communication difficulties are not often identified as the precipitating cause in malpractice suits, they are widely believed to be the major predisposing cause.

Experts on malpractice have concluded that what happens in the office, and the kinds of relationships that are developed there, are critical in setting the stage for a patient's subsequent reaction if there are problems in treatment. In one of our own studies, we found that the visit communication of primary care physicians with a history of malpractice differed from those who had never been sued; sued doctors, in contrast to those who had never been sued, spent less time, were less likely to use humor in their visits, and were less likely to solicit patients' opinions about care or check that patients understood information (Levinson, Roter, Mullooly, Dull, & Frankel, 1997). In a similar vein, Hickson and colleagues (Hickson, Clayton, & Entman, 1994) found that patients of physicians with prior malpractice claims (but who were not involved in the suits) had twice as many complaints about their care than patients of doctors who had not been sued. The patients' complaints included such things as feeling rushed, ignored, receiving inadequate explanations or advice, and spending less time with the doctor during routine visits.

It is believed that the majority of malpractice claims would not be pursued if the patient, or the patient's family, were not angered over failures or disappointments in the patient's relationship with the physician. The kinds of complaints mentioned above appear to make their way into legal documents. A study of complaints that actually appeared in malpractice depositions revealed that communication problems were present in 70% of the reviewed cases (Beckman, Markakis, Suchman, & Frankel, 1994).

THE DYNAMIC NATURE OF DOCTOR-PATIENT RELATIONSHIPS

Expectations regarding medical authority and patient autonomy are complex, they are often unstated, and they are dynamic. The patient's social world, physical condition, stage and type of illness, and a host of cultural and demographic factors, have relevance for the kind of relationship a patient desires. As these conditions change, the kind of relationship that works best for a patient may change. It is easy to suggest that doctors and patients should choose one another by "relationship fit" meaning that a consumerist patient will be happiest with an egalitarian and accommodating physician, or a patient who prefers to defer to the physician is best served by a "take-charge" doctor. However, there are structural and situational constraints that limit the freedom of patients to change doctors at will, or for physicians to easily dismiss their responsibilities to patients (Haug & Lavin, 1981). Because of economic constraints or the nature of an unusual medical condition, the doctor and patient may be more deeply committed to one another, and for far longer, than either would like.

But, perhaps a more compelling argument for negotiation and accommodation rather than discontinuity, is the likelihood that needs and circumstances will change over time, and that the relationship could better serve both its parties if it had the flexibility to change as well.

3

Thinking Critically and Creatively in the Conception, Conduct, and Interpretation of Medical Communication Research

The study of doctor-patient communication is difficult and complex. However, there is also a richness and depth to the human experience addressed in this work that excites, delights, surprises, and engages us far more than what we could have envisioned some 25 years ago when we began our own studies. In an effort to make the research task more understandable, we have devoted this chapter to a discussion of key theoretical, methodological, and measurement issues that we have considered in our work. These issues are important in their own right, but they will also provide a foundation for the remaining chapters that deal with substantive questions about the conduct and interpretation of medical communication research.

Our starting point is the often-voiced lament that research on provider-patient communication is not "theoretical enough." We point out several ways in which the theoretical value of research can be brought out and developed (J. A. Hall & Schmid Mast, 2004). Next, we outline some of the key methodological challenges facing researchers as they consider the design and conduct of communication research. Finally, we address the longstanding and intense debate concerning the paradigmatic distinctions between quantitative and qualitative approaches to the assessment of medical dialogue.

THINKING THEORETICALLY

Often, research on provider-patient communication is criticized for not being sufficiently "theoretical." Granting agency review panels, journal editors and reviewers, and members of the investigator community can often be heard to voice this lament, both on and off the record. Consider the following statements:

> Although considerable attention has been given to doctor-patient communication, relatively little research on this topic is grounded in theory. (Cegala, McGee, & McNeilis, 1996, p. 1)

> The literature concerning doctor-patient communication is abundant and comprehensive . . . [but] the main characteristics of the field are diversity and fragmentation. Part of the problem is the lack of a unifying theoretical framework to enable integration of models and to guide application of the research findings. (Frederikson, 1993, p. 225)

> An underestimated problem in research on doctor-patient communication is the influence of a-theoretical decisions on concrete research. (Ong, de Haes, Hoos, & Lammes, 1995, pp. 905–906)

Statements such as these clearly suggest that the literature on provider-patient communication may be descriptively adequate but is superficial and devoid of meaning. But what, exactly, is the deficiency? And, when people make this allegation, are they all talking about the same thing? The vague and imprecise demand to be more theoretical is not helpful to researchers. Though it is true that there exists no overarching theory for why things happen as they do between doctors and patients, nevertheless we are not as pessimistic as some authors are in interpreting this as a marker of banality. The field of medical communication is still young, and there are many complicated processes and many variables to consider (personal, situational, organizational, behavioral, emotional, physiological, etc.). Because it is not a laboratory science, there will always remain more ambiguity and more unanswered questions than we might wish. Although the field is blossoming, both in terms of theoretical understanding and in the development of practical, useful advice for physicians and patients, progress can be more rapid and advances more dramatic if the concept of "being theoretical" is expanded to include more than deriving research hypotheses from established theories or developing a new theory oneself.

Theories can vary greatly in their breadth, complexity, and other dimensions. For our present purposes, we will consider a theory to consist of a set of conceptual (and potentially operationalizable) constructs for which the author states the causal interrelations. In other words, a theory is an attempt to explain empirical phenomena at a conceptual level. In our view, there are several ways in which one may engage in theoretical thinking.

The first way to think theoretically is to *ground one's research hypotheses with a clear rationale for what one is looking for and why.* One way to do this is to derive a hypothesis from an established theory. As an example, cognitive dissonance theory (Festinger, 1957) states that the experience of holding contradictory thoughts creates an unpleasant need to resolve the contradiction, especially if one has freely chosen the underlying behaviors. From this, one can derive the prediction that choosing or remaining with a particular provider is likely to make the patient see that provider in a favorable light. So, it is not surprising that public opinion polls show that people are far more critical of the character and competence of doctors in general than they are of their own doctors, commonly rating their own doctors as being above average. Since not all doctors can be above average, at least some patients must be exaggerating their doctors' virtues. This sounds a lot like the Lake Woebegone phenomenon, in which all the children are above average. This is an example of using a theory to understand a common (possibly irrational) judgment.

Much research that one might call atheoretical is actually grounded in theory but the author has failed to explicitly develop the arguments (hypotheses, predictions, rationales, etc.) that would make the theoretical grounding clear. Such research can be called latently theoretical: the theoretical basis for the work could be brought to light if the author made the effort to do so. The theory on which a piece of research is grounded need not be an existing, named theory in order to be considered valid. An investigator could very well ground his or her research on a homegrown theory, or even just a novel point of view from which justifiable hypotheses can be developed. Good hypotheses need not be deduced from a formal theory; they can come from the researcher's own experience, from common beliefs or observations, or from the desire to reconcile conflicting empirical results (Rosenthal & Rosnow, 1991). But, regardless of where a hypothesis comes from, good theoretical grounding requires good *theorizing*: the author must provide adequate background and logical justification for the proposed research and its hypotheses.

Another way of thinking theoretically is to develop an *optimal study design.* Even without identifying any existing theory, research can be made more theoretical if the design or mode of analysis is chosen specifically to advance causal understanding of a phenomenon and thereby to help develop or improve a theory. Randomized experiments (randomized controlled trials) are theoretical in this sense, because such studies are designed to demonstrate cause and effect. It is important to note, however, that a randomized experiment can still be theoretically lacking if the researcher does not offer compelling reasoning behind the predictions, provides inadequate interpretations of the results, or does not discuss mediating processes—the "black boxes" that invariably lie between manipulated independent variables and measured dependent variables. An investigator conducting a randomized experiment will not always be able to address a black box empirically (i.e., measure potential intermediate steps in the causal process), but he or she should always speculate about it. When research is specifically designed to capture mediating processes, its theoretical value increases dramatically.

Another way to think theoretically is to *apply a theory to the interpretation of the findings*, that is, to give careful thought to what the findings mean. The author may use the findings to help settle a theoretical question, may compare the findings to previous findings, may discuss alternative interpretations of the findings, or may use the findings to develop a coherent new idea about some phenomenon or process. Thus, research interpretations can be theoretical by producing new amendments to an existing theory, new ideas for future research, and new generalizations.

Finally, theoretical thinking includes an *appreciation of impact*. Often, one responds to a piece of research with the feeling that it is (or is not) "theoretically interesting." What does this mean? Such a reaction often refers to the feeling of impact in its several forms. The reader can be intellectually or emotionally stimulated; the results might be surprising or huge in magnitude; or the study might be particularly ambitious, addressed to an especially important question, designed in an especially original way, or written in such a way that it gets the reader thinking (either in favor of the idea or against it). The feeling of impact can also be related to the anticipation of the research's importance in the real world or potential for the advance of scholarly understanding. Thus, we believe that the "not theoretical enough" criticism is often a way of saying "not interesting enough."

THINKING METHODOLOGICALLY

Establishing Cause and Effect

Conducting research that documents the interactions between doctors and patients is understandably difficult. It is done in the real world with people who have pressing, serious business to attend to, and it is often done in large, busy, and complex organizations such as hospitals. Permission is required at several levels of bureaucracy, the approval of human-participants boards is required, and the permission of the providers and patients themselves must be obtained. The time required to assemble a team of researchers as well as to cultivate the cooperation of the staff can be enormous. The monetary costs required for personnel to arrange the study, gather the data, and analyze the data are high. If audio or video recordings are done, the costs of applying coding schemes to quantify the data, or to produce and analyze written transcripts of the dialogue, can be astronomical. On top of that, doctors and patients cannot usually be imposed on for much of their valuable time.

Sometimes it seems like a miracle if even a simple study can get off the ground, not to speak of a study that can address big, complex, and important questions in an airtight manner.

Though many studies have been done that somehow managed to overcome various obstacles, it is still the case that compromises have to be made. It remains very difficult to conduct studies in which the circumstances of care (including the behaviors of the physicians or patients) are experimentally manipulated. Such an experimental approach is crucial to understanding what causes what. Physicians are understandably reluctant to let researchers tell them how to behave, for this seems like a terrible invasion of their professional prerogatives. Nevertheless, without properly randomized studies, it is extremely difficult to determine whether their behaviors are helpful, harmful, or neutral in impact.

Sometimes it is argued that randomly assigning people to different experimental interventions or treatment groups, as is required to determine cause and effect, may be unethical, either because the decision maker is not allowed free choice, or because people in one group will be deprived of the innovative treatment that the other group receives. These arguments make sense only if the treatment or innovation is known to be beneficial and for whom it is beneficial. However, if this were known, there would be no need to do the research. We conduct experimental research precisely because we do not know the impact of the treatment. Under this circumstance, the *only* ethical course is to use chance—that is, random assignment—to determine who is exposed to the treatment. Of course, the investigator must hold the sincere (and defensible) belief that the experimental treatments are likely to be beneficial.

Mostly, research on physician-patient interactions is correlational, rather than experimental, meaning that we can determine whether variables are related to each other, but we may be very unsure of which causes the other, or even whether either does cause the other. To illustrate the problem, in a large review of studies of patient satisfaction with medical care, it was found that only 14% were randomized studies in which variation in satisfaction could be traced to a certain cause (J. A. Hall & Dornan, 1988a). Sometimes, the researcher is able to measure additional variables that might be producing or influencing the correlation in question, and then remove the influence of those variables statistically. Doing this provides somewhat more confidence about what's going on, but only up to a point. Mostly, researchers are left to spin stories about causal factors (usually stories they personally favor). To make matters worse, most journals do not allow space for authors to go into long discussions about all the possible meanings that their correlations might have. Consider the following example: If patient satisfaction is correlated with how much information the doctor provided to the patient, does this mean that getting information makes the patient satisfied? Or does this mean that being satisfied makes the patient behave in a way that inspires the physician to tell more? Or do these effects build on each other in a spiraling fashion? Or is some third variable responsible for both satisfaction and information provision? All too often, authors offer only very simple explanations or none at all.

It is obvious that more experimental research is needed in the study of doctor-patient communication. Certainly, in the early phases of investigating a research question, correlational studies are desirable for establishing the plausibility that causal paths are present. But, after a certain point, a correlation will be well established (as many have been), and it is time to move to experimental studies, not only to ascertain what is really causing what, but also to understand the intervening or mediating variables in the process.

Looking for Moderators

Regardless of whether the research is correlational or experimental, the relation between two variables is unlikely to be the same irrespective of how, when, where, and in whom they are measured. Therefore, researchers need to look for variations in personal and situational characteristics that are associated with different magnitudes of effect; in other words, researchers need to look for moderator variables. If a researcher determines, for example, that emotional support from a provider has a stronger relation to satisfaction among cancer patients than among healthy people having an annual checkup, the researcher has uncovered a moderator (having cancer or not) (Baron & Kenny, 1986). This would be an important finding, but, we must point out, one that has its own causal ambiguity because a moderator is usually not itself an experimentally manipulated variable. Therefore, one might not be able to say exactly what caused this difference in strength of effect. In the example given, does emotional support better predict satisfaction in cancer patients because oncologists deliver emotional support better than other physicians do? Because cancer patients value emotional support more than other patients? Because the cancer patients were older, and older patients are easier to please? Because the cancer patients were women, and women especially value emotional support? Because the cancer patients' emotional issues were different from those of other patients, and some emotional issues are easier to talk about or resolve than others? This example clearly illustrates how complex the interpretational dilemmas can be for the researcher. Ideally, the research would be designed at the outset to examine these different possibilities.

So far, in studies of doctor-patient communication, the documentation of moderator effects is in its infancy. Mostly, we do not even know when they exist, much less how they should be interpreted. Two studies of what is supposed to be the same question may show different results because of random sampling error (sometimes called the "margin of error") and not because the results truly differ. Or, if the results do actually differ, it may be hard to figure out which study characteristics are responsible.

Meta-analysis, or the quantitative analysis of multiple studies, is a method that allows one to surmount some of these difficulties (Hedges & Cooper, 1993). By amassing all of the available studies on a topic and applying statistical techniques, the researcher can often determine whether a moderator is at work and what that moderator is. To give hypothetical illustrations of moderators that could be uncovered through meta-analysis, one might find that a given drug is especially effective for patients in a certain age group, that one way of talking to patients about adherence to their pill regimen works better than another way, or that nurses are more effective in providing patient education than doctors are.

As it stands, researchers are often not able to explain why studies contradict one another. But, as more studies accumulate, the chances of understanding the operation of moderator variables is greatly increased.

Is the Use of Standardized and Analogue Patients Valid?

Although it is difficult to argue with the value of authentic settings for observational studies, the contribution of simulation to our understanding of medical dynamics is worthy of consideration. This is especially evident when patients and physicians are under extreme stress and when observational techniques designed to capture the intense dynamics of the situation may risk disruption of care. In these circumstances, we might worry about manipulating or interfering with the care of actual patients in a manner that may have an unintentional or unanticipated negative impact—particularly in terms of psychological distress and burden. In the oncological setting, the study of bad news delivery may present these challenges. There are also important, but rare, circumstances worthy of investigation that may simply be logistically impossible to investigate in natural settings. The study of physician communication detailing a medical mistake to his or her patient, for instance, may be an example of an infrequent incident with critical significance. Finally, it may be impossible to disentangle predictor variables that often covary, such as patient race, socioeconomic status, and gender, when trying to untangle their separate effects, even with large databases and sophisticated statistical techniques (McKinlay, Lin, Freund, & Moskowitz, 2002).

For these reasons, some circumstances may demand the creative use of standardized and analogue patients in addition to, or instead of, actual patients. Use of the standardized patient, a person trained to simulate a patient's illness in a standardized way, has become increasingly accepted, over its 30-year history, as a method of instruction and evaluation of medical trainees and as a powerful and flexible research tool (Ainsworth et al., 1991; Barrows, 1993). Many of these studies have noted the behavior of physicians in standardized patient encounters to be highly realistic and often indistinguishable from their behavior with actual patients.

Analogue patients are distinct from standardized patients in that they are usually untrained subjects who are recruited to imagine (through role-playing) that they are the patient depicted in some medical circumstance, often with provider or communication attributes that are experimentally manipulated. The circumstance may be as simple as a written vignette or as complex as actual or simulated videotapes of medical encounters. In this way, the analogue patients provide researchers with a proxy for actual patient perceptions or judgments (Roter, Hall, & Katz, 1987). Physicians may also be recruited in a parallel manner to act as analogue physicians, physicians who imagine that they are the physician depicted in the medical circumstance, to provide a proxy for clinical judgments and professional behaviors under experimentally manipulated conditions (McKinlay et al., 2002; Schulman et al., 1999).

Evidence that standardized patient encounters are realistic and that analogue patients are sensitive to variations in physician performance (even when with standardized patients) is available in a number of studies. For instance, the impact of physicians' task-oriented and socioemotional behaviors when interacting with standardized patients was evaluated by presenting audiotapes of these visits to analogue patients who rated the sessions for satisfaction, recall of information, and affective impressions of the physician (Roter et al., 1987). The analogue patients clearly distinguished the task-oriented behaviors from the socioemotional behaviors of the physicians, and the analogue patients showed a pattern of association linking these behaviors to satisfaction and recall of transmitted information.

The well-cited study by Schulman and colleagues (1999) illustrates the use of varying actor characteristics (race, gender, age, and social class) in standardized performances to investigate the independent effect of identity characteristics on physicians' clinical decision making. The results illustrated the role of nonmedically relevant patient characteristics, particularly the patient's race and gender, in influencing physicians' test-ordering behavior. McKinlay and colleagues (2002) have further used this methodology to assess the impact of physician characteristics on clinical decision making. In that experiment, the investigators concluded that the physician's medical specialty, and the physician's race and age, had an unexpected and nonmedically relevant effect on the physician's clinical decision making when presented with a standardized videotape performance of a patient presenting medical symptoms.

Other examples, specific to the complex and emotionally charged communication of oncology, are also convincing. Shapiro and colleagues randomly assigned 40 women who were at risk for breast cancer to view one of two videotapes of an oncologist presenting mammogram results (Shapiro, Boggs, Melamed, & Graham-Pole, 1992). The information in both videos was identical, and the mammogram results were described as "ambiguous," but in one tape the oncologist appeared worried. Those viewing the nonworried oncologist correctly recalled significantly more information than those viewing the worried doctor, and the viewers of the worried oncologist evidenced increased heart rate, as well as higher scores on pen-and-paper measures of anxiety. Though the oncologist in the videotaped disclosure of the mammogram results did not discuss the severity of the illness, patients in the "worried" group believed that the situation was more severe. In a second study along similar lines, Fogarty, Curbow, Wingard, McDonnell, and Somerfield (1999) found positive effects, evident to analogue patients, from the inclusion of a brief expression of compassion into a videotaped simulation in which an oncologist confirmed the bad news that a patient's breast cancer had metastasized. In that study, a compassion manipulation of approximately 40 seconds of dialogue in a 17-minute video, during which the physician touched the patient's hand and reassured her that she was not alone and that the physician would "be there" for her, significantly reduced reported anxiety among analogue patients and had a generally positive influence on their ratings of the physician's compassion and partnership characteristics.

An important implication from this stream of research is the powerful effect of simulations in inducing experimental realism in analogue patient and analogue physician raters. The most important methodological implications of these studies are (1) that experimental use of standardized patient performance can be effective in inducing realism, as reflected in analogue patient and physician ratings, and (2) that standardizing the patient's performance is useful in factorial experimental designs to disentangle the independent and combined contributions of characteristics that often covary (e.g., race, gender, and social class) in studies of outcomes, such as patient judgments or clinical decision making.

Whom Should We Study?

Reviews of medical communication research clearly demonstrate that physicians are studied far more frequently than any other type of health care provider. Not only are nonphysician providers largely ignored in this literature, but visit companions (family members or friends present during the medical visit) are commonly excluded from communication analysis, irrespective of their presence in the medical encounter and the role they may play in shaping the medical exchange (Roter, 2000a). Consequently, the majority of communication studies assess medical communication largely as a monologue from the perspective of the physician, and, occasionally, what an individual patient may say back. It is with good reason, then, that it has been argued that communication research in the medical context has been myopically focused on the communication of physicians (Kreps, 2001).

This does not, however, necessarily imply that our knowledge of physician communication is exhaustive. A critical assessment of the literature, as reviewed in the upcoming chapters, suggests that much of what is known of provider communication is based on what is said during the delivery of outpatient care by primary care physicians who are primarily Caucasian males (L. A. Cooper & Roter, 2003). Even when diversity in the provider population is present, there is little attempt to disentangle the independent effects on communication of key identity characteristics, such as gender and race, from one another or from contextual variables, such as specialty training and practice experience. This has resulted in diminished attention to the important independent and interactive role that identity characteristics play in shaping the nature and dynamics of communication (McKinlay et al., 2002).

Furthermore, the majority of communication studies assess medical exchange from the perspective of the physician, rather than as a dialogic exchange between interactants. And, even when communication is assessed as a reciprocal and interactive phenomenon with two participants, it almost always consists of the exchanges of a single patient with his or her primary physician. As discussed in Chapter 4, there are only a few empirical studies on how companions affect the dynamics of medical exchanges, and virtually all of these studies have been conducted within the context of geriatric visits. The frequency with which companions accompany oncology patients to their medical visits is likely to be much higher than those reported for routine geriatric exchanges. Indeed, many oncologists suggest that patients invite a spouse or other family member to be with them during medical visits in which critical information is conveyed and treatment decisions will be made; the role of the companion(s) is generally to provide both emotional and instrumental support for the patient (Baile et al., 1999).

QUALITATIVE AND QUANTITATIVE APPROACHES TO INTERACTION ANALYSIS

A wide variety of approaches to the qualitative assessment of patient-physician interactions is evident in the literature; several of these approaches reflect particular theoretical and methodological roots and use formalized transcription and analytic guidelines (Mishler, 1984; Sacks, Schegloff, & Jefferson, 1974). The three primary formalized approaches are discourse analysis, conversational analysis, and narrative analysis. Although there is a good deal of overlap, discourse analysis approaches tend to focus on how talk within medical interactions changes, establishes, or maintains social/power relationships, while conversational analysis approaches tend to address the structural features of talk (e.g., turn-taking rules and question-and-answer sequences) that obligate participants to pursue certain courses of action. Narrative analysis approaches tend to focus on the stories of participants' experiences (Roter & McNeilis, 2001). Other approaches are more ad hoc in nature and idiosyncratic in their methods (Roter & Frankel, 1992). Nevertheless, the common ground shared across all qualitative approaches is the preservation of the verbatim record of spoken dialogue in the participants' own words.

There are many different quantitative communication-assessment instruments represented in the literature. A recent review of the area identified a total of 44 different instruments used (Boon & Stewart, 1998). Approximately one-third of these were designed to evaluate the performance of medical students in communication skills training programs; of these, only three were used by an investigator other than the system's author, although none of these have been used within the past 15 years. The review also identified 28 different systems used for assessment of communication in research studies. However, only four of these systems were used by multiple investigators, including those of Bales (1950), Stiles (1992), Roter and Larson (2002), and Stewart et al. (1995).

A brief overview of each of these four systems is provided here.

Bales's Process Analysis System

Concerned with group dynamics, Bales (1950) developed an analysis scheme for assessing the problem-solving and decision-making processes of small groups. In applications of the method to medical encounters, Bales's scheme has been substantially modified in a variety of ways, including the application of the scheme to dyadic exchange. Bales's method categorizes problem-solving processes as belonging to one of two domains: the emotionally neutral, task-focused domain, or the largely socioemotional domain. An interaction is described as falling into one of 12 mutually exclusive categories; six categories are conceived as affectively neutral and ascribed to the task dimension (e.g., making a suggestion or asking for orientation), and six categories are viewed as representing the socioemotional dimension of communication, which is divided into positive and negative affective categories (e.g., agreeing or disagreeing, and showing tension release or showing tension).

Analysis using Bales's method is based on transcripts of the verbal events of the encounter that are operationally defined as the smallest discriminable speech segments to which the rater can assign classification. A unit may be as short as a single word or as long as a lengthy sentence; compound sentences are usually divided at the conjunction, and sentence clauses are scored as separate units when they convey a single item of thought or behavior, such as an acknowledgment, evaluation, or greeting. Inasmuch as Bales's system was originally devised as a method for studying group interactions, many researchers who derived theoretical direction from the system substantially changed the substantive categories to more directly reflect dyadic medical interactions. Nevertheless, the first studies of medical dialogue in which Bales's process analysis system was applied (in the late 1960s and 1970s) are still cited as the seminal studies of doctor-patient communication (Freemon, Negrete, Davis, & Korsch, 1971; Korsch, Gozzi, & Francis, 1968).

The Verbal Response Mode (VRM)

Another theoretical approach, based on linguistic theory, was introduced by William Stiles: the verbal response mode (VRM) system (Stiles, 1992). Like Bales's system, the VRM taxonomy is a general-purpose system for coding speech acts and consequently is not specific to medical encounters. The unit of analysis is a speech segment (similar to Bales's system), defined grammatically to be equivalent to one psychological unit of experience, or a single utterance.

The system forms a taxonomy that implies a particular interpersonal intent or microrelationship between the communicator and the recipient. There are three principles of classification: the source of experience, operationalized as attentive (to the other speaker) or informative (speaker's own experience); presumption about experience, operationalized as directive (controlling dialogue) or acquiescent (deferring to the other's viewpoint); and, finally, the frame of reference, defined as presumptuous (presuming knowledge about the other person) or unassuming (not presuming particular knowledge). Each of these classification principles is dichotomous, taking the value of either "the speaker" or "the other." The taxonomy bases the assignment of language segments on the following categories: disclosure, edification, advisement, confirmation, question, acknowledgment, interpretation, and reflection. Using this taxonomy, each speech segment is coded twice, once with respect to its grammatical form, or literal meaning, and once with respect to its communicative intent, or pragmatic meaning. Thus, there are 64 possible form-intent combinations—eight pure modes in which form and intent coincide, and 56 mixed modes in which they differ.

The VRM has been used by its author and others in studies in the United States, the United Kingdom, and the Netherlands. These studies include those of patients in primary care, cancer treatment, and psychiatric treatment (Stiles, 1992).

Roter Interaction Analysis System (RIAS)

The RIAS is explicitly designed to reflect medical exchange and is derived loosely from social exchange theories related to interpersonal influence and problem solving (Roter & Larson, 2002). It provides a tool for viewing the dynamics and consequences of patients' and providers' exchange of resources through their medical dialogue. The social exchange orientation is consistent with health education and empowerment perspectives that view the medical encounter as a "meeting between experts" that is grounded in an egalitarian model of the patient-provider partnership that rejects expert-domination and passive-patient roles.

A useful framework for organizing and grounding RIAS-coded communication in the clinical encounter is the functional model of medical interviewing (Cohen-Cole, 1991). Task behaviors fall within two of the medical interview functions: "gathering data" to understand the patient's problems and "educating and counseling" patients about their illnesses and motivating patients to adhere to treatments. Affective behaviors generally reflect the third medical interview function of "building a relationship" through the development of rapport and demonstrating responsiveness to the patient's emotions. A fourth function of the visit can be added, "activating and partnership building," to enhance patients' capacity to engage in effective partnerships with their physicians. Although not explicitly defined by the authors of the functional model, the use of verbal strategies to help patients integrate, synthesize, and translate between the biomedical and psychosocial paradigms of the therapeutic dialogue deserves special note. The "activating" function facilitates the expression of patients' expectations, preferences, and perspectives so that they may more meaningfully participate in treatment and management decision making (Roter, 2000a).

The RIAS is applied to the smallest unit of expression or statement to which a meaningful code can be assigned, generally a complete thought, expressed by each speaker throughout the medical dialogue. Unlike most other systems, coding is usually done directly from audio or videotape, bypassing the use of transcripts. The coding units are assigned to mutually exclusive and exhaustive categories that reflect the content and form of the medical dialogue. Form is used to distinguish statements that are primarily informative (information giving), persuasive (counseling), interrogative (closed- and open-ended questions), affective (social, positive, negative, and emotional), and process oriented (partnership building processes, orientations, and transitions). In addition to using form, content areas are specified for exchanges about medical conditions and histories, therapeutic regimens, lifestyle behaviors, and psychosocial topics that relate to social relations and feelings and emotions.

In addition to the verbal categories of exchange, coders rate each speaker on a 6-point scale that reflects a range of affective dimensions, including anger, anxiety, dominance, interest, and friendliness. These ratings have been found to reflect voice tone channels that are largely independent of literal verbal content (J. A. Hall, Roter, & Rand, 1981). The system is flexible and responsive to the study context because it allows for the addition of tailored categories. Coders may also mark the phases of the visit so that the opening, history segment, physical exam, counseling and discussion segment, and closing are specified; this allows communication that falls within these parts of the visit to be analyzed and summarized separately.

The RIAS system has been used widely in the United States and Europe, as well as in Asia, Africa, and Latin America; it has been used in primary care settings, in oncological practice, in specialty practice, and even in veterinary medicine. An annotated list of more than 150 RIAS-related studies is available on the RIAS Web site (https://rias.org).

Patient-Centered Measure (Stewart)

Developed specifically to assess the behaviors of patients and doctors according to the patient-centered clinical method (McWhinney, 1989; M. Stewart et al., 1995), a method of scoring the "patient-centeredness" of audiotaped or videotaped medical encounters was developed (Brown, Weston, & Stewart, 1989; Levenstein, McCracken, McWhinney, Stewart, & Brown, 1986; M. Stewart et al., 1995). The scoring procedure is described in detail elsewhere (Brown, Stewart, & Tessier, 1995; Henbest & Stewart, 1989; M. Stewart et al., 1995); briefly, scores range from 0 (not at all patient-centered) to 100 (very patient-centered) based on assessment of three main components. The first component is "understanding of the patient's disease and experience" (statements related to symptoms, prompts, ideas, expectations, feelings, and impact on function). Every pertinent statement (as many as are applicable), for each of the six elements, made by the patient is recorded verbatim on the coding sheet. The coder assigns a score to the statement as to whether the physician provided preliminary exploration (yes or no) or further exploration (yes or no), or cut off discussion (yes or no). The second component, "understanding the whole person," explores the context of a patient's life setting (e.g., family, work, social supports) and stage of personal development (e.g., life cycle). The third component is "finding common ground" (mutual understanding and agreement on the nature of the problems and priorities, the goals of treatment and management, and the roles of the doctor and patient).

The patient-centered method has been most often applied in primary care and used in assessment of medical student and physician performance (Stewart, 1995).

THINKING QUALITATIVELY AND QUANTITATIVELY

A debate of longstanding intensity concerning the assessment of medical dialogue centers on the distinction between quantitative and qualitative approaches (Roter & Frankel, 1992). The heat of the debate comes not merely from a disagreement over the relative advantages and disadvantages of qualitative and quantitative methods, but from the broader perception that these approaches reflect incompatible paradigms. Advocates of each of these methods have not only argued their own relative merits, but have maintained unusually critical and intellectually isolated positions.

A well-recognized list of attributes distinguishes the quantitative and qualitative paradigms and their adherents. The quantitative world view is characterized as hypothetico-deductive, particularistic, objective, and outcome oriented; its researchers are logical positivists. In contrast, the qualitative world view is characterized as social anthropological, inductive, holistic, subjective, and process oriented; its researchers are phenomenologists (Reichardt & Cook, 1969). An allegiance to a particular paradigm not only implies a worldview, but also a paradigm-specific method of inquiry and even styles of presentation.

The extension of the qualitative and quantitative paradigm controversy to evaluation of medical dialogue has been made by several authors. Quantitative approaches have been characterized as reflecting the biomedical model's emphasis on the scientific method and the translation of observations into numbers. These researchers present statistical summaries and correlates of "objectively" measured patient and provider behaviors. Qualitatively inclined researchers, on the other hand, rarely assign numerical values to their observations, but prefer instead to record data in the language of their subjects, almost always presenting actual speech through verbatim transcripts of audio and videotape recordings.

As noted elsewhere (Roter & Frankel, 1992), the paradigmatic perspective which promotes mutual exclusivity is in error; we see no inherent logic to the limitations established by tradition, other than tradition itself. Indeed, we have noted that there is a certain parallelism between the systems of open-sea navigation described by the cultural anthropologist, Thomas Gladwin, and the debate among researchers of the medical encounter over qualitative and quantitative methods (Gladwin, 1964). The system of navigation represented by the European tradition is distinguished by the plotting of a course prior to a journey's beginning that subsequently guides all decisions regarding location. The extent to which the journey "stays the course" is a testament to the navigator's skill. The Islanders of Truk face the problem of managing long distances over uncertain conditions in a very different manner than the Europeans. The Trukese navigator has no pre-established plan of any kind; rather, experience from previous voyages and information at hand during the current sailing trip account completely for Trukese navigational expertise.

Much of the debate in medical interaction research has focused on comparing methods independent of particular contexts, questions, or outcomes. Although it is quite clear that the methods used by Gladwin's navigators differ in both kind and degree, it is also the case that they both solve the same practical problem successfully. The value of Gladwin's analysis is that it includes both context and outcome as determinants of methodological utility. As well, it raises a caution about attempts to understand one set of methodological practices in the terms used to describe another. The presence or absence of map-making skills is essentially irrelevant to the Trukese navigator, as is the ability or inability of European navigators to read local wave patterns.

Methods of research, like those of navigation, are open to description in their own terms, and should be judged on the extent to which they succeed in answering the questions which they raise in the context in which they were raised. And, each approach has shortcomings. The time-consuming nature of qualitative analysis prohibits its application to large databases, and sometimes the researcher's close reading and interpretation of the discourse can raise questions about subjectivity and reliability. Quantitative analysis, relying more on surface characteristics (e.g., frequency counts or ratings) rather than deep meaning, can seem superficial and atomizing in its measurements (for example, by counting up how many questions were asked altogether) so that moment-to-moment continuity and sequence can be lost. But this is not necessarily so; sequential analysis is possible by coding behavior within segments of the medical visit, or by maintaining a record of real time so that exchanges can be characterized in terms of what behavior tends to follow what behavior, and when. Superficial though the quantitative analyses may seem to some, this disadvantage may be offset by the much higher level of evidentiary certainty gained by conducting inferential statistics on the data.

Rather than choosing one approach or the other, creative researchers can combine both approaches within the same study, either in separate phases of the analysis or by developing quantitative indicators that capture some of the richness that is the hallmark of qualitative analysis. An example would be to have neutral raters read or listen to the conversation and make quantitative, thematic assessments that allow the rater to make a complex inference about the speaker's intention or state—for example, how intense the patient's misgivings about a given procedure seem to be, or how much the patient appeared to be persuaded by the physician's arguments, rated on a rating scale. As long as such judgments pass the test of inter-rater reliability, they would permit a quantitative treatment of psychologically rich (i.e., qualitative) information.

Thus, respect for alternative methods does not preclude combining methods to maximize discovery and insight. The potential of a new paradigm, representing a qualitative and quantitative methodological synthesis, is exciting; the extent to which this synthesis will have an impact will be a function of its practical utility and relevance to the theory and practice of medical interviewing over time.

4

The Influence of Patient Characteristics on Communication between the Doctor and the Patient

It has been argued that the basis of trust between patients and their physicians lies in the physician's dedication to "universalism," that is, the responsibility to treat all patients alike without regard to particular attributes or ascribed traits (Parsons, 1951). It is reasoned that patient care must be universalistic or suspicion and caution would prevail over trust and confidence in the doctor-patient relationship. Fear that physicians might act upon ageist, class-related, or racist stereotypes could undermine the fabric of the social contract upon which the therapeutic relation rests. For vulnerable populations, with few resources and little political or social power, the consequence of disparities in the delivery of care is evident in health itself—high levels of disease morbidity and a reduced life expectancy. Indeed, the Institute of Medicine's report "Unequal Treatment" has made the investigation of factors related to variations in health care delivery a public health research priority (Smedley, Stith, & Nelson, 2003).

There are at least four mechanisms by which one might hypothesize physician behavior to relate to patient characteristics. First, there may be an unintended association between the care process and patient attributes that is produced by mutual ignorance of social or cultural norms. The differences that exist between physicians, who are largely well-educated, middle-class Caucasians, and patients who are not may lead to very basic communication difficulties. For instance, citing sociolinguistic theorists, Waitzkin (1985) generalized to the medical context the finding that middle-class subjects tend to be verbally explicit while working-class subjects tend to communicate more implicitly through nonverbal signals. Waitzkin suggests that physicians may

not be attuned to the nonverbal signals of working-class patients and may easily miss or misinterpret patient requests for information or cues of distress.

A second possible pathway through the medical care process may be
affected by patients' sociodemographic characteristics; physicians may
be consciously, and quite appropriately, addressing the varying responses
to illness that socially patterned expectations for care demand. These
needs reflect the diverse attitudes, beliefs, and expectations of the groups
to which a patient belongs (J. G. Fox & Storms, 1981). For instance, in his
classic study of ethnicity and pain, Zborowski (1952) found that patients'
interpretations of pain and expectations regarding pain control varied
widely across ethnic groups and that these expectations were communicated
to physicians. In this case, tailoring pain management effectively maximized
medical care.

A third explanation is the possibility that physicians' behavior is elicited,
in some cases even demanded, by the patient. The reciprocation concept
that we discussed earlier in this book applies here. Much of what a person
does in interaction is in response to a triggering behavior by the other person. Thus, emotional tone tends to be reciprocated in kind, and many dis-
crete behaviors occur in complementary sequences such as questions
followed by answers. Therefore, if physicians' behavior is correlated with
patients' attributes, it can stem from the physicians responding to patients'
behaviors that are correlated with patients' attributes.

Finally, it is possible that physicians, like others in our society, are negatively affected by stereotypes. Physicians have generally scored about the
same as nonphysicians in surveys reflecting attitudes toward the elderly or
the poor (Marshal, 1981; Price, Desmond, Snyder, & Kimmel, 1988) and
appear to share the same negative stereotypes about physically unattractive
people as does the society at large (Nordholm, 1980). Further, the range in
physicians' political and ideological beliefs indicates a broad spectrum of
response to patient groups (Waitzkin, 1985). Physicians' negative attitudes
or the assumptions they make about a patient's personality, motivation, or
level of understanding clearly have implications for the care they give.

In this chapter we will explore the extent to which patient characteristics
such as age, gender, social class, ethnicity, health status, and physical
appearance affect doctor-patient communication.

AGE

It has been maintained that ageism, the system of destructive false beliefs
about the elderly, is pervasive in our society and is reflected in the health
context through negative physician attitudes, lack of respect for the autonomy and decision-making abilities of the elderly, and a general reluctance

to deal with older patients (Greene, Adelman, Charon, & Hoffman, 1986; Haug, 1981).

There is evidence from the investigation of nonverbal or paralinguistic qualities of interaction to suggest that communication between elderly patients and providers, at least in nursing homes, differs from that of communication between younger patients and providers. Caporael (1981) focused on the use of displaced baby talk to the institutionalized elderly. Baby talk is a simplified speech pattern with distinctive paralinguistic features of high pitch and exaggerated intonation contour that is usually associated with speech to young children. More than 22% of speech to residents in one nursing home was identified as baby talk. Further, even talk from caregivers to the elderly that was not identified as baby talk was more likely to be judged as directed toward a child than was talk between caregivers. The investigators concluded that this phenomenon is widespread and that baby talk directed toward elderly adults was not a result of fine tuning of speech to individual needs or characteristics of a particular patient, but rather a function of social stereotyping of the elderly. The interpretation of these findings, however, may carry some caveat. The investigators also studied whether baby talk was perceived positively or not by nursing home residents. It was found that when baby talk was stripped of its context and content filtered so that the words could not be understood, it sounded more comforting, less irritating, and less arousing than adult talk. When rated in context, however—that is, when played to judges who were themselves institutionalized elderly—preference was related to functional ability: the lower the elderly judge's functional ability, the more positively the baby talk was rated (Caporael, Lukaszewski, & Culbertson, 1983).

Evidence of negative physician attitudes toward the elderly adults in outpatient medical practice is sparse and somewhat contradictory. From an affective perspective, physicians were judged to be significantly less positive; observers listening to audiotapes of the visits rated physicians as less egalitarian, patient, engaged, and respectful when talking with older patients (Greene et al., 1986). These investigators found little evidence of blatant ageism in their analysis of the study audiotapes, but did find some differences in how topics were addressed, the emotional tone of the visit, and several patterns of exchange that were related to patient age. More medical topics and fewer psychosocial issues were discussed in interviews with older patients, and, further, when older patients raised psychosocial issues, doctors tended to be less responsive than when younger patients raised similar issues. Physicians were rated higher regarding the degree of questioning, information provided, and support given to younger compared to older patients. In additional analysis, the investigators reported that agreement on the major goals and major medical topics discussed during the medical visit was significantly greater for younger patients and their physicians than for older patients (Greene, Adelman, Charon, & Friedmann, 1989).

Also concluding that visits with elderly patients may carry more tension than those of younger patients, Stewart (1983) found that physicians were less likely to engage in "tension release" (joke and laugh) when with older patients and that older patients were much more likely to express antagonism or defensiveness than younger patients.

In contrast, other studies have found some communication advantage for older patients. Hooper, Comstock, J. M. Goodwin, and J. S. Goodwin (1982) found physicians to be more courteous with elderly compared to younger patients, particularly those patients over the age of 74. Similarly, other research has found evidence of greater warmth directed toward the "old-old," that is, to patients over the age of 74 (Roter, 1991). Older patients have also been found to receive more explanations, more explanations in nontechnical and comprehensible language, and more explanations that were matched to the sophistication of the question than younger patients (Waitzkin, 1985).

It should be noted the above studies are all correlational in nature and that older age is associated with a number of factors that may explain, at least in part, its observed relationship with communication. Among these are poorer health status (discussed later in this chapter) and the presence of a visit companion during the medical visit. Estimates vary, but it seems that from one-quarter to one-half of geriatric primary care patients are accompanied by a companion during their medical visits (Prohaska & Glasser, 1996; Schilling et al., 2002). Moreover, the presence of a companion increases with patient age and declining health status (Clayman, Roter, Wissow, & Bandeen-Roche, 2005). Based on a handful of studies, companions who accompany patients during their routine medical visits are most often the patient's spouse or an adult child and, less frequently, a nonrelative friend or paid caretaker (Clayman et al., 2005; Fortinsky, 2001). Despite the frequency of companions, there has been relatively little descriptive study of how their presence or actions may influence the medical decisions patients make or the care they receive. Nevertheless, some researchers fear that the intrusion of a third party into the doctor-patient relationship may result in a loss of patient autonomy and jeopardize confidentiality (Clayman et al., 2005).

There is some evidence that patients tend to be more passive in their medical visits and decision making when a companion is present. Greene et al. (1986) found that elderly patients raised fewer topics and were less assertive and expressive when accompanied than in visits without companions. Moreover, accompanied patients were sometimes excluded from the conversation between a companion and physicians, and physicians directed information toward the companion, rather than the patient (Beisecker 1989;

Greene, Majerovitz, Adelman, & Rizzo, 1994). Other behaviors that may be interpreted as undermining the patient were also observed. Hasselkus (1988), for instance, reports that companions may take on an information-giving role in the visit, sometimes contradicting the patient or disclosing information the patient had not wanted revealed.

The presence of a companion has also been described as beneficial to the care process: physicians give more information when family members are present than when patients are alone (Labrecque, Blanchard, Ruckdeschel, & Blanchard, 1991; Prohaska & Glasser, 1996) and report that the presence of a companion increases both patient and physician understanding of one another (Schilling et al., 2002). In a detailed observational study of companions during routine geriatric visits, Clayman and colleagues described a variety of communication behaviors—including those that can be regarded as helpful to the care process, as well as those that may not be (Clayman et al., 2005). Companions assisted both the patient and the physician in understanding one another; they helped the patient by asking the doctor clarifying questions and repeating the doctor's explanations to the patient in layman's terms, and they helped the doctor better understand the patient by clarifying elements of the patient's history and bringing up pertinent medical topics. Companions also facilitated patient involvement in the medical visit by asking the patient clarifying questions, prompting the patient to discuss topics of importance, and by asking for the patient's opinion and preferences. Companions engaged in a variety of controlling behaviors, as well, including answering for the patient, interrupting the patient, or discussing their own health problems or occasionally attempting to ally with the physician to influence the patient to do something that either the physician or companion wanted the patient to do.

More than half of the companions (52%) in the Clayman study engaged in at least one positive behavior and no controlling behaviors, 41% engaged in at least one behavior of each kind, and no companions engaged in controlling behaviors in the absence of positive behaviors. Companions of sicker patients appeared to be especially active and assisted both the patient and the doctor in understanding one another, as well as facilitating patient involvement in care. Facilitation of patient involvement in care had an especially positive effect; patients were more than 4 times as likely to be active in decision making if their companions facilitated their involvement than if they did not play this kind of role (Clayman et al., 2005).

We know little about moderating effects such as the visit companion's ethnicity, culture, and age cohort, and about the nature of familial relationships on communication dynamics. An intriguing question is the effect on communication of having "baby boomers" as companions in the medical visits of their aging parents, compared with spouses or contemporaries acting as visit

companions. We might speculate that these adult children bring an assertiveness to their medical encounters that can dominate the visit and perhaps
contribute to a verbal withdrawal by the patient from the medical dialogue
(as described by Greene et al., 1986, above); alternatively, the presence
of a consumerist companion may spur assertive behavior on the part of
some patients as implied by the finding that patients with facilitating companions are more active in decision making.

GENDER

Although almost everyone is intrigued by differences in male and female
behavior patterns, medical care researchers have not given this topic much
attention until recently. And, although a typical study will have ample numbers
of male and female patients, it will not typically have ample numbers of
male and female physicians; usually the physician sample is small and at
least two-thirds of the physicians are male. Therefore, the crucial question
of how physician and patient gender interact in shaping the process of care
is hard to address. Nevertheless, the available literature on patient gender
offers some thought-provoking findings. (Results related to physician gender are discussed in Chapter 6.)

The effect of gender on health care use is evident at even a young age.
Lewis and colleagues (C. E. Lewis, M. A. Lewis, Lorimer, & Palmer, 1977)
investigated this question by establishing a procedure within a Los Angeles
elementary school whereby children aged 5 through 12 were permitted to
leave the classroom and seek out the nurse without approval of their teacher.
Before the study, boys and girls had about the same number of visits to the
nurse, but, after 2 years, their patterns of use were virtually identical to
those of adults. Children from more affluent backgrounds made more visits,
and girls came more often than boys. For each visit a boy made to the nurse,
girls made 1.5 visits, virtually identical to the gender ratio for adults who
are 35–54 years of age (1.55 female visits for each male visit).

In a study focusing on patient gender differences in communication,
Waitzkin (1985) found that female compared with male patients were given
more information and that the information was given in a more comprehensible manner, that is, technical explanations were also explained or
reworded in simpler language. There was also a tendency for physicians to
appropriately match their response to female patients' questions in terms of
technical sophistication, consequently avoiding the appearance of talking
up or talking down to them (Waitzkin, 1985). In an analysis of the same
data set, Wallen and associates (Wallen, Waitzkin, & Stoeckle, 1979) demonstrated that the greater amount of information given to women was
largely in response to women's tendency to ask more questions in general

and to ask more questions following the doctor's explanation. Very similar conclusions were drawn by Pendleton and Bochner (1980) in their British study of general consultations. These investigators found that female patients were given more information than males and that this information was in answer to their more frequent questions.

Research of ours on routine medical visits at a large teaching hospital did not find that female patients obtained more information overall. However, they had more medical/technical jargon addressed to them and they gave more information of a medical nature to the doctor than male patients did, perhaps in reciprocation of receiving more technical language. Females were also more explicit than male patients in making sure that they understood the physician by paraphrasing and interpreting his or her statements and checking that the physician understood what they had said (J. A. Hall, Irish, Roter, Ehrlich, & Miller, 1994a).

Several other investigators have reported that female patients receive more positive talk and more attempts to include them in discussion than males. Stewart's analysis of primary care practice found that physicians were more likely to express "tension release" (laughter, mainly) with female patients, and were also more inclined to ask them about their opinions or feelings (Stewart, 1983). Female patients returned laughter in their visits, but male patients appeared more likely to take the initiative in exchange. For instance, male patients showed higher scores on a "patient-centered" cluster of behaviors that included giving suggestions, opinions, information, and orientation to the physician, as well as more negative verbal behaviors, including disagreements and antagonisms. Another study of some 150 patient visits reported by Hooper et al. (1982) similarly concluded that female patients had more positive experiences with their physicians than male patients. Information giving was significantly higher, and there was greater use of empathy with female compared to male patients. Physicians were also less likely to interrupt the visit by leaving the room when with female compared to male patients.

One of our large studies (J. A. Hall & Roter, 1995), involving over 600 routine medical visits, found that male and female patients made the same number of statements but that these differed in emotional tone. Women made more statements of concern, as well as agreements and disagreements, and had voices that were rated as more anxious and interested. In other words, female patients had a more emotionally expressive style. In a reciprocal pattern, the physicians addressed more emotionally concerned talk and more disagreements to women. When the patients were asked after the visit what kind of physician they preferred, women said they preferred a "feelings-oriented" over a "thoughts-oriented" physician. Thus, the style of communication addressed to female and male patients could be seen to match the patients' stated preferences.

Although there are studies that fail to find an association between patient gender and aspects of communication, none showed less information given to female patients. As noted by Hooper et al. (1982), communication differences attributable to the patient's gender may reflect sexism in medical encounters, but this may act to the advantage of female patients, as they have a more informative and positive experience than is typical for male patients. Many studies in nonmedical settings have shown differences in male and female communication styles. It is not unreasonable to expect that these differences may also show up in how doctors and patients act toward each other. In general, the interpersonal style of women is more engaged, warm, and immediate than that of men (J. A. Hall, 1984; J. A. Hall, 2006). The sexes differ in their use of smiling, facial expressiveness, gazing, interpersonal distance, angle of facing another person, touch, and bodily gestures—with women in each case showing a behavior pattern that suggests more accessibility and friendliness. Women emit more "back channel" responses such as nodding and saying "uh-huh," "yeah," and "I see," behaviors that serve to encourage the other's speech and signal attentiveness. Women often find it easier to disclose information about themselves in conversation (Dindia & Allen, 1992).

Women and men differ in their communication skills, both overall (B. R. Sarason, I. G. Sarason, Hacker, & Basham, 1985) and in terms of nonverbal communication in particular (J. A. Hall, 1984). Women decode the meanings of nonverbal cues better than men do (e.g., facial expressions, tone of voice), and they express emotions more accurately through nonverbal cues than men do. Communication involving female patients (or female patients and female doctors) may be more effective in terms of factual information exchange as well as the more subtle aspects of understanding the doctor's feelings and intentions. There is evidence that women are more proactive as patients; for example, among patients with chronic disease, women are more likely to prefer an active role in medical decision making than men (Arora & McHorney, 2000), and women both report (Kaplan, Gandek, Greenfield, Rogers, & Ware, 1995) and have been observed to experience (Gotler et al., 2000) more opportunity for decision making in their relations with their doctors than men. In the Kaplan et al. study, patient participation in decision making was particularly low when male patients interacted with male physicians.

People also treat the sexes differently—for example, by gazing and smiling more at women than at men, and sitting or standing closer to women than to men. Differential treatment of the sexes may reflect a particular affinity for one's own gender, or disregard or disrespect for another. In our study of 100 internal medicine visits, physicians (who were evenly divided between males and females) used voices with a more bored, calm, and submissive tone when addressing female patients (Hall et al., 1994a). Although the voice tone findings could indicate that physicians were tuning out female patients, an alternative interpretation is that physicians' less active and less dominant manner with females simply reflects a more low-key manner of interaction. This would be consistent with nonclinical research that finds voice tone addressed to males to be the most business-like, condescending, and dominant (J. A. Hall & Braunwald, 1981).

Together, these patterns suggest that women interacting with women are the most immediate nonverbally, while men interacting with men are the least so (J. A. Hall, 1984). Our recent analysis of effects of physician gender on patient communication suggests that gender concordance appears to strengthen many of the gender effects described in this chapter (Roter & Hall, 2004). A more detailed discussion of gender concordance on medical communication is presented in Chapter 6.

SOCIAL CLASS, CULTURE, AND ETHNICITY

In one of the first studies of the relation of health to social class and culture, Koos (1954) found not only that recognition of serious symptoms differed among the classes but that the social evaluation of the symptoms differed. For instance, Koos found that working-class women often suffered from persistent backaches but rarely sought medical care for them. Further, these women felt that undue attention to so common a condition would inspire ridicule rather than sympathy. In contrast, women of higher social class were much more likely to rate persistent backache as a serious symptom deserving medical attention.

A second process may also be at work. Some symptoms and social roles may be mutually supporting, that is, some symptoms may be seen as evidence of especially good or dedicated performance. For instance, in a study with graduate students, Zola (1966) found that tiredness was often recorded in symptom diaries but infrequently noted as a reason for concern. For these students, fatigue meant they were working hard and was taken as an indication of doing the right thing. Consequently few students saw persistent fatigue as a reason for seeking medical help, even though they were well aware of the host of quite serious medical and psychological conditions often associated with it. Fatigue became something to be proud of, and to talk about, rather than a cause of concern. While conducted some 40 years ago, the sentiment expressed by Zola's graduate students is still evident, at least in some graduate programs!

While studies reflect the impact of social class on the definition of what symptoms are noteworthy and how these symptoms will be presented to the physician, ethnicity and cultural background also show similar effects. A classic study of health and ethnicity (Zola, 1963) found that, among patients seeking medical care from several different outpatient clinics, those of Italian rather than Irish or Anglo-Saxon descent were much more likely to be labeled as having "psychiatric problems" by their physicians, despite the fact that there was no objective evidence that these problems were more frequent among them. When the doctors could not identify any specific disease to explain the patient's symptoms, which happened equally often in each of the ethnic groups, Italians almost always had their symptoms attributed to psychological problems, whereas this almost never happened in the case of the Anglo-Saxons and Irish. Differences were evident, however, in how the Italians presented their chief complaints. Italians reported more pain, more symptoms overall and in more bodily locations, and more consequent dysfunction including interference with their social and personal relations.

From these findings, the investigator speculated that the Italians and Irish have ways of communicating illness that reflect different ways of handling problems within the culture itself. The Italians tend toward drama and exaggeration as a means of dissipating and coping with anxiety, whereas the Irish have a tradition in which control and denial are foremost (Barzini, 1965). This became evident in the very different ways these patients presented their symptoms to their doctors. Similar findings were reported by Zborowski (1952) in describing ethnic variations in response to pain. Anglo-Saxon patients viewed pain in an "objective" and rather unemotional way, the Irish often denied pain, and Italian and Jewish patients were highly emotional and exaggerated in their expressions of pain. Moreover, the Italian patients sought immediate relief from pain and were satisfied as soon as the pain ceased, but the Jewish patients were more concerned about the significance of their pain for future health and resisted pain medication for fear that it would mask a significant symptom.

Not only was the way in which patients presented their pain significant, but appropriate treatment was tied to this expression. Pain killers were effective for the study's Italian patients, but not for the Jewish patients until reassurances about future health were also provided. Only a physician sensitive to these distinctions could appropriately recognize these patient needs. A follow-up study, using the same clinics as in the Zborowski study some twenty years later (Koopman, Eisenthal, & Stoeckle, 1984), found similar differences between Anglos and Italians in how pain was reported; however, the effect of patient ethnicity was most evident with patients over 60 years of age. Patient gender was also found to be important in this study, with pain being most likely to be reported by older female Italians and least likely to be reported by older male Anglos. For younger patients, now second and third generation in this country, the process of acculturation had diminished the ethnic effects.

Given the correlation between social class and ethnicity in our society, it is not surprising that doctors' treatment of patients in different ethnic groups tends to parallel their treatment of patients in different social classes. A number of studies have documented lower levels of information given to patients of low socioeconomic status, and correspondingly higher levels of patient diffidence in the presentation of symptoms, question asking, and overall levels of verbal activity (Bain, 1979; Pendleton & Bochner, 1980; Waitzkin, 1985). An explanation for these social class differences has been suggested by Waitzkin (1985), who described the sociolinguistic culture of the working class as tending to be less verbal than that of the middle class. Because of the tendency away from direct (verbal) communication, working-class patients may be communicating their desire for information in ways that physicians are likely to miss. Doctors, like other members of the middle class, expect communication to be verbal and explicit; if patients have questions, they expect that the patients will ask those questions. Consequently, nonsolicited information is not offered and reticence is taken as an indication of lack of interest.

This effect may also be present in the communication of patients belonging to ethnic minorities. Reviews of the literature show that Caucasians receive care that is of higher interpersonal quality than Blacks or Hispanics receive, as well as more positive talk and more information, even within the same medical practices (e.g., Bartlett et al., 1984; Epstein, Taylor, & Seage, 1985; J. A. Hall, Roter, & Katz, 1988; Hooper et al., 1982; van Ryn, 2002). For example, one study found that African American patients received fewer recommendations for open-heart surgery, although they had equal clinical need, and of all the patients who received such a recommendation, African American patients had surgery less often (Maynard, Fisher, Passamani, & Pullum, 1986). One hypothesis regarding this outcome is that the discussions with minority patients regarding surgical options are less extensive, informative, or effective in helping patients make clinically appropriate decisions. In another study, physicians demonstrated more skillful use of questioning, facilitation, and empathy when talking with Anglo American patients as compared to Spanish American patients (Hooper et al., 1982). The investigators suggested that poorer physician performance was particularly evident in communication skills requiring listening when talking with minority patients.

We believe that negative stereotypes of disadvantaged social groups affect the way doctors interact with patients. We also believe this is largely unintentional and that doctors are only dimly aware of how their stereotypes may influence their behavior, if at all. Like most people, doctors probably attribute any differences they do notice in their own behaviors to the character, aptitude, or needs of the other (in this case, the social class or minority status of the patient). When one's own behavior can be construed as negative, a person is particularly inclined to blame it on the other person. But, as discussed earlier in this book, behavior has many sources, and a negative attitude held by a doctor is only one source. Other examples we have given include the reciprocation of behavior directed by the patient toward the doctor (e.g., the reciprocation of emotional qualities in nonverbal behavior; J. A. Hall, Roter, & Rand, 1981) and response to actual demands made by the patient (e.g., women get more information because they ask more questions; Wallen, Waitzkin, & Stoeckle, 1979). Additionally, differences in health needs may alter communication because doctors may have to reallocate their behaviors given the reality of inflexible patient schedules. In a later section we discuss health status as an illustration.

LITERACY

As highlighted by a recent Institute of Medicine report, nearly one-quarter of the American public is functionally illiterate and another one-quarter is only marginally literate (Nielson-Bohlman, Panzer, & Kindig, 2004). The problem of poor literacy and its significance to patient care is made more meaningful when put within the health context. Using a functional literacy measure designed to reflect tasks common to the health context—for instance, reading prescription drug labels, appointment slips, tests and procedure preparation instructions, and giving informed consent to a routine procedure—Baker and colleagues demonstrated that fully one-third of the patients who were admitted to their inner-city hospital were unable to perform these basic tasks (D. W. Baker et al., 1996). These findings are consistent with earlier research reporting inadequate or marginal functional health literacy to be as high as 35% among English-speaking patients and 62% among Spanish-speaking patients seeking care at public inner-city hospitals. The prevalence of low literacy skills among elderly patients (more than 60 years of age) was even higher, averaging 80% for both English- and Spanish-speaking patients (M. V. Williams, Baker, Parker, & Nurss, 1998).

Because low literacy levels are so common, physicians are likely to routinely encounter patients with limited literacy skills. Nevertheless, physicians are largely unaware of their patients' literacy deficits. In one study by Bass and colleagues, fewer than 10% of patients reading below the sixth-grade level were identified as having a literacy problem; a full 90% of the patients with a reading deficit were unrecognized by their physicians (P. F. Bass, Wilson, Griffith, & Barnett, 2002). A second study, by Lindau and colleagues, with women attending an obstetric and gynecology clinic or a women's HIV clinic, also found low levels of resident physician awareness of their patients' literacy problems, with accurate recognition limited to about one-quarter of the patients with inadequate reading skills (Lindau, Tomori, McCarville, & Bennett, 2001).

Low levels of recognition are not surprising. Consider the results of Parikh and colleagues who report that one in three patients who were identified as having low literacy skills denied any difficulty reading or understanding what they read (Parikh, Parker, Nurss, Baker, & Williams, 1996). This suggests that these patients may not even be aware themselves of the extent of their limitations or are unwilling to admit these limitations to a researcher. Among those patients in the study who did admit having trouble reading, 40% revealed feelings of shame and more than half of these patients had never told their spouses or children about their reading difficulties. Notably, 75% of the patients with a literacy deficit reported that they never mentioned their limited literacy skills to their physicians.

This finding is consistent with findings from focus group discussions of poor readers in which serious and widespread communication difficulties with doctors were revealed (D. W. Baker et al., 1996). Patients complained that they felt they were neither listened to nor adequately informed about their medical problems and treatments in ways they could understand. Despite this frustration, few patients asked questions or otherwise revealed their reading difficulties to their physician. Most simply did not think this was something the physician would be interested in knowing.

Several studies have described the relationship between patients' educational level and medical communication. It should be noted that the common measure of education, years of schooling completed, reflects educational exposure—not achievement. Adult reading comprehension tends to be 2 to 5 years below reported levels of education completed. Moreover, a patient's socioeconomic status, age, and ethnicity may all influence the magnitude of the gap between exposure and achievement. Davis and colleagues found this gap to be almost 5 years when low-income minority patients were examined but only half as pronounced, 2.6 years, when Caucasian, middle-income patients were studied (Davis, Crouch, Wills, Miller, & Adebhou, 1990).

Despite these caveats, several studies have documented a relationship between education and medical communication. Better educated patients, and patients of higher socioeconomic backgrounds, received more physician time, more total explanations, and more explanations in comprehensible language than other patients (Waitzkin, 1985). Ironically, physicians not only gave more information to these patients, but they also appeared to go out of their way to offer these explanations in clear, nontechnical language. Multivariate analysis of these data further demonstrated that the patient's level of education was more important than social class, in general, in explaining information transmittal. Waitzkin concluded that the educational aspect of social class is a particularly strong factor in doctor-patient communication. In a similar vein, Stewart (1983) reported that better educated patients were much more likely to receive a justification for their treatment regimens from their physicians than were less educated patients.

For patients in the Stewart study, more information came at a price; the better educated patients received less emotional support from their physicians than did those patients without some university-level training. The opposite finding in regard to emotional support, however, was reported in several studies of pediatric visits wherein better educated parents of patients received more emotional support than less educated parents. The classic study by Korsch and associates (Korsch, Gozzi, & Francis, 1968) of pediatric encounters in an emergency walk-in clinic found that better educated parents of patients were more likely to express their fears and hopes to the doctor and that they had a better chance of having these responded to or dealt with than less educated parents. Similarly, the pediatric study by Wasserman and associates (Wasserman, Inui, Barriatua, Carter, & Lippincott, 1983) found that better educated mothers received more reassurance, encouragement, and empathy during pediatric visits than less educated mothers. Finally, C. E. Ross and Duff (1982) observed indicators of performance quality, both technical and interpersonal, in over 400 pediatric visits and reported that poorly educated parents received worse care on all accounts from their physicians. Also noted in this study was that low-income families did not have as consistently negative experiences as did the children of the poorly educated. Thus these authors concluded, as did Waitzkin (1985), that education has more significance for health experience than other socioeconomic indicators.

Direct examination of the communication dynamics of patients with low literacy levels and their experiences in medical visits has been largely limited to small studies (Roter, 2004). An exception is a recent study by Schillinger and colleagues (Schillinger et al., 2003; Schillinger, Bindman, Wang, Stewart, & Piette, 2004). The health literacy levels of over 400 English- and Spanish-speaking diabetic p atients were assessed and these scores were related to the patient's rating of the quality of communication with their doctor in the past 6 months using a standard measure of interpersonal communication. The investigators found that inadequate functional health literacy was associated with a lower quality of interpersonal processes of care across three of seven communication dimensions, including general clarity, explanations of conditions, and explanations of processes of care. The relationship between literacy and these communication quality ratings were even stronger after statistically adjusting for a variety of confounding variables, including whether the patient's primary language was English or Spanish, whether the physician spoke Spanish, the duration of the patient-physician relationship, and a variety of socio-demographic and health status measures.

Fortunately, the recall deficits associated with low literacy are remediable. In analyzing audiotape data from his study, Schillinger further found that, when physicians addressed cognitive issues by assessing recall and comprehension of new concepts introduced during the medical visit, patients were more likely to have hemoglobin A1c levels below the mean, compared with patients whose physicians missed the opportunity to clarify and reinforce important information (Schillinger et al., 2003). The recall and organizational problems associated with poor literacy may be especially exacerbated in older individuals who are simultaneously suffering cognitive and physical decline. The dramatically low levels of literacy found among many elderly populations is likely a reflection of both actual literacy deficits but also cognitive decline associated with procedures such as open heart surgery, chemotherapy, and kidney dialysis, as well as common chronic conditions such as hypertension and diabetes (D. W. Baker et al., 2002). It is reasonable to speculate that the effect of cognitive decline appears earlier and is even more devastating for patients with low literacy levels than others since they are likely to have fewer cognitive compensatory resources.

In summary, we can say that physicians engage in more dialogue, and are more informative, with better educated and more literate patients. Moreover, the evidence suggests that education may play a key role in the differential communication to patients of varying socioeconomic groups. Because of the confounding of socioeconomic status, education, and race in our society, some of the observed disparity in the delivery of care to minority group patients may also be, at least partially, explained in this way. It has long been known vulnerable populations have trouble finding health care and get less of it. Now it appears that the problems of these groups are not entirely structural and that they suffer poorer treatment even after they gain access to the health care system. Although worse health for these groups has usually been assumed to stem from lifestyle factors such as stress or poor nutrition, or from difficulties in getting care, the possibility must also be raised that disadvantaged patients may be sicker partly because of the way in which they and their doctors communicate.

HEALTH STATUS

Physicians seem to like their healthier patients more than their less healthy ones (J. A. Hall, Epstein, DeCiantis, & McNeil, 1993; J. A. Hall, Horgan, Stein, & Roter, 2002). This relation was found regardless of whether health was defined in terms of social, emotional, or functional criteria, or was rated overall by the patient, and even when standard patient sociodemographic characteristics were controlled for. We believe this to be a disturbing result, and one which may come as a surprise to physicians, who probably believe they find the more challenging cases to be most stimulating and rewarding. Though this may be true in certain cases, the more prevailing fact of routine medical practice is that many medical conditions are chronic and therefore do not offer the rewards of a cure nor the variety and excitement of an acute condition. Thus, the frustration and the repetitiveness associated with treating patients with chronic conditions may reduce physicians' liking for them.

Some of this effect may also come from the patient's side. Patients with a chronic or hard to diagnose condition may cease acting appreciative; after all, they are not getting cured and indeed may be on a downward slide. Also, patients who feel ill are likely to be grumpy, unresponsive, and possibly even unwashed or unkempt, and patients whose distress is of an emotional nature may be particularly erratic or unrewarding in interpersonal interaction. Research has documented that sicker patients behave more negatively (J. A. Hall, Roter, Milburn, & Daltroy, 1996). Thus, it is not too surprising if physicians have more feelings of liking for their patients in better condition. However understandable a physician's reaction may be, the implications are considerable. One common finding from numerous studies on patient satisfaction is that sicker and more distressed patients are less satisfied with their care, as summarized by J. A. Hall, Feldstein, Fretwell, Rowe, and Epstein (1990). Sicker patients also like their doctors less (J. A. Hall et al., 2002). The dissatisfaction of sicker patients could stem from the generally negative outlook likely to be held by a person in physical or mental distress, but it could also stem from negative cues given off by the physician.

There is evidence that dissatisfied patients are dissatisfied with other things too—with government, community, and other nonmedical aspects of their everyday life. Being sick may color their views about the world, meaning that their dissatisfaction with medical care may have little to do with the care per se. But the nature of their medical care could play a part in the dissatisfaction of sicker and more emotionally distressed patients. Considering that doctors like sicker patients less, it is possible that doctors treat sicker patients in a dissatisfying manner.

These two hypotheses were pitted against each other in two studies that supplied the necessary measures of satisfaction, health status, and communication process (J. A. Hall, Milburn, Roter, & Daltroy, 1998). The most prevalent finding was that the sicker patients' lower satisfaction was not brought about by physician behavior. However, in one of the studies, the physicians appeared to be implicated in their sicker patients' dissatisfaction. Physicians curtailed social conversation with sicker patients, which was then shown through statistical modeling to be predictive of lower satisfaction.

Apparently, the patients valued some amount of social conversation and resented its absence. From this study, we do not know whether physicians curtailed social conversation because of their lower liking of the sicker patients, or because they pragmatically decided to devote more of the visit to these patients' more complex health problems. Either way, a negative spiral could be triggered that would only work to the further detriment of the patient's well-being.

ATTRACTIVENESS AND LIKING

Addressing the influence of physical appearance on doctor-patient communication, Hooper et al. (1982) rated the physical appearance of the patients included in their observational study. Patients who appeared rumpled, disheveled, or whose clothing looked dirty had encounters in which the physician was less likely to use appropriate open-ended questions, to elicit details, and to allow the patient an opportunity to ask questions. There were similar effects on the quality of nonverbal communication, including eye contact, the physician's body position, and observers' ratings of courtesy. Patients with the highest ratings on appearance—those who were "clean and pressed" in a three-piece suit or attractive dress, and had their hair clean and neatly styled—had fewer physician-initiated interruptions during their visits than other patients. These findings are quite similar to the negative experience reported for patients of lower socioeconomic or ethnic minority backgrounds, as well as patients in a worse state of physical or mental health.

That physicians like some patients more than others is clearly implied in discussions of the hateful patient (Groves, 1978). Hateful patients are those who appear to physicians as overly dependent, demanding, manipulative, rejecting, or self-destructive. Groves suggested that the negative reactions these patients evoke from their physicians should be used as clinical data to facilitate better understanding and more appropriate psychosocial management. But while physicians are trying to turn their negative feelings to good use, they should also be alert to the fact that their degree of liking will probably leak out and be detected by the patient. Indeed, physicians and patients both have a significant (though not great) degree of accuracy in judging how much each likes the other (J. A. Hall et al., 2002).

Though physicians may be uncomfortable with the suggestion that their personal liking of patients makes a difference in the care they provide, it is probable that the medical visit, like any other interpersonal encounter, is influenced by approach and avoidance tendencies on the part of both physician and patient. Though there is not much work focusing specifically on liking, there is a great deal of indirect evidence to suggest that liking matters in medical visits. First, whenever a study shows that doctors treat patients of different types differently, one must ask whether group stereotypes are translating into degrees of liking and disliking for whole categories of patients. Research that asks physicians for their attitudes and beliefs about various groups such as male and female patients, "difficult" versus "easy" patients, physically attractive versus unattractive patients, and patients of different social classes does suggest that physicians' attitudes vary across such groups (Bernstein & Kane, 1981; Biener, 1983; Dungal, 1978; J. A. Hall et al., 1993; Leiderman & Grisso, 1985; Nordholm, 1980; Smith & Zimny, 1988).

CONCLUDING THOUGHTS

There are certainly differences in doctor-patient communication that may be attributable to differences in such patient characteristics as gender, age, race, educational level, and social class. What is not clear from the body of literature reviewed is whether these distinctions are uniformly negative in their effect on patient care. In regard to gender, for instance, in contrast to the widely publicized view that medical care is given in a way that disparages or discriminates against women, sexism may work in favor of better medical care for female patients. This is consistent with utilization studies that have established that females receive more services than males, including return visits, tests, and prescriptions (Verbrugge & Steiner, 1981; Weisman & Teitelbaum, 1989). Beneficial treatment for the elderly is less clear; older patients may receive more information and perhaps courtesy than others, but it may be communicated in a manner that undermines autonomy and active participation in medical exchanges. Less conflicting evidence has been found in regard to the experience of patients of lower social class backgrounds, minorities, and the poorly educated—these patients have more negative health experiences than others.

There appears to be evidence for all four earlier hypothesized mechanisms by which patient characteristics may affect doctor-patient communication. There may be unintended violations of universalism due to miscommunication, with the poor and poorly educated not making their desire for information clear to physicians. There may be varying physician response to socially and culturally patterned expectations and attitudes toward evaluation of symptoms and pain management. Under some circumstances, physicians may be responding directly to patient elicitation, for instance more question asking by female patients leading to more information directed towards female compared with male patients. And, finally, violations of a universalistic orientation through stereotypes, dislike, and prejudice may occur in interaction with unlikable or "difficult" patients, and perhaps the poorly educated, the poor, and minority patients.

We hope it is clear from our discussion in this chapter that we do not claim that communication deficiencies are entirely a matter of doctors' attitudes and have nothing to do with how different kinds of patients behave. An articulate, college-educated patient is likely to make different demands of his or her physician than a poorly educated and verbally diffident immigrant. But because these patients' psychological and physical needs may be exactly the same, doctors cannot base their responses entirely on the patient's initiatives. Unfortunately, for a doctor to see past immediate demands and try to fathom patient agendas that may be unexpressed may require more patience and sensitivity than many harried doctors, with their minimal training in interpersonal skills, are willing to muster.

Although the social class, education, and ethnicity of patients cannot be changed, providers' behaviors might change if both they and their patients became more aware of how these characteristics intrude upon the provision of medical care. This would be a first step toward assuring that the social contract between patients and their doctors is honored.

5

The Influence of Physician Characteristics on Communication between the Doctor and the Patient

The doctor's identity in terms of personal character and personality, as well as sociodemographic and cultural background, has relevance for how patients are treated and the kind of medicine that will be practiced. This chapter will explore the question of whether there is such a thing as a definitive "doctor-type" and what the implications are for physician deviation from expectations in this regard. We will explore how individual characteristics of the student relate to their chances of selection into medical school, training experience, specialization, and the way they are likely to treat their patients. Because of the influence of physician gender on communication, and the dramatic rise over the last decade in the number of women in medicine, we have devoted a separate chapter, Chapter 6, to that discussion.

PHYSICIAN ETHNICITY

With the exception of gender, changes in the traditional demographic profile of medical students have been modest, particularly when viewed in terms of underrepresented American minority groups, including Native Americans, African Americans, Mexican Americans, and Mainland Puerto Ricans (Barzansky, Jonas, & Etzel, 2000). Despite small gains in minority student enrollment in the 1990s, enrollment has remained flat over the past 10 years, at about 5% for African American students and 3.5% for Hispanic students.

African Americans currently constitute less than 10%, and Hispanics some 6%, of the medical school applicant pool (R. A. Cooper, 2003). While the number of African American applicants is expected to remain constant over the next two decades, the number of Hispanic applicants is expected to rise by 50% (to 9%), even as Hispanic Americans are projected to account for 22% of the U.S. population (R. A. Cooper, 2003). The situation for applicants of Asian ancestry is different. In 2000, Asian Americans accounted for 18% of medical applicants, far out of proportion with the 4% of the U.S. population that they comprise. While representative of an ethnic minority, Asian Americans are not considered an underrepresented minority group.

Studies have shown that African American physicians are more likely to provide health care to African American patients than are their Caucasian counterparts (Bach, Pham, Schra, Tate, Hargraves, 2004; Xu et al., 1997). The extent to which racial matching occurs is documented in a recent study of over 4,000 physicians and 150,000 African American and Caucasian Medicare beneficiaries (Bach et al., 2004). African American patients were 32 times more likely than Caucasian patients to see African American physicians (22.4% versus 0.7%). Nevertheless, it should be kept in mind that most patient visits—both African American and Caucasian—are to Caucasian physicians. There is no doubt that at least some part of this utilization pattern is due to minority patients' sensitivity to communication difficulties in their medical visits, some of which is attributed to the ethnicities of their physicians. For instance, a study of patients in the Detroit Area found that a higher percentage of African American than Caucasian patients reported less visit time allocated to them (35% versus 46%) and lower levels of physician respect (47% versus 64%) (Malat, 2001). In a similar vein, a nationwide survey of patient attitudes toward medical care found that African American patients were almost twice as likely as their Caucasian counterparts (16% versus 9%) to report being treated with disrespect during a recent health care visit. African American patients were also more likely than Caucasians (23% versus 16%) to report one or more measures of poor communication with their physician (i.e., problems understanding the doctor, feeling that the doctor did not listen to them, or having but not asking questions) (Collins et al., 2002).

Minority patients' reports of physician conduct are substantially different if their physician is of the same ethnicity (Chen, Fryer, Philips, Wilson, & Pathman, 2005; Saha, Komaromy, Koepsell, & Bindman, 1999). Also based on a national surveys, Saha and colleagues (1999) found that overall satisfaction was higher and ratings of respect, explanations, listening, and accessibility were significantly more positive for those African American and Hispanic respondents who had a physician of the same ethnic background. An interesting caveat to these findings was suggested by Chen and colleagues: preference for, and higher satisfaction with, a physician of the same ethnicity, among both African American and Hispanic patients, was associated with strong beliefs about racial discrimination in health care (Chen et al., 2005).

It is interesting to note that communication difficulties are not limited to minority patients in the U.S. Ethnic minority patients in the Netherlands, primarily immigrants from Eastern Europe and former Dutch colonies, have also reported more problems in their relationships with Dutch practitioners and less satisfaction with the communication of their visits than Dutch patients (van Wiernigen, Harmsen, & Bruijnzeels, 2002).

Despite the communication difficulties suggested in the studies described above, there has been little direct (observational) research on the communication impact for minority patients of having a physician of the same ethnicity. An exception is our own recent study in which audiotapes of minority patients in race-concordant and race-discordant visits were analyzed (L. A. Cooper et al., 2003). The study included 142 African American patients and 110 Caucasian patients receiving care from 31 physicians (of whom 18 were African American and 13 were Caucasian) in 16 urban primary care practices.

Race concordance was related to several aspects of the visit process. Both African American and Caucasian patients in race-concordant encounters had visits that were on average two minutes (10%) longer than patients in race-discordant encounters, even after adjustment for factors known to be associated with longer patient visits (older age, higher socioeconomic status, and poorer health status). The race-concordant visits were also characterized by slower speech speed and perhaps a lessened sense of time urgency. As noted in the Malat study above, visit duration may have particular salience for African American patients because they report shorter visits and lower satisfaction with time spent when in race-discordant relationships with physicians.

In addition, race-concordant visits received higher global ratings of positive affect from observers. The significance of positive affect may reflect feelings of social or racial group affiliation, enhanced trustworthiness, greater respect, or positive expectations. These attributions are likely to influence both the communication process and patient judgments of such things as how much their doctor likes them. It is interesting to note a striking similarity in the race-discordant findings to those of the Dutch study mentioned earlier in which ethnic minority patients reported more communication difficulties when seeing Dutch physicians than did Dutch patients (van Wiernigen et al., 2002). Their examination of visit audiotapes found that the communication between ethnic minority patients and their Dutch doctors, compared with Dutch patient visits, were characterized by lower global ratings of patient and physician friendliness, lower ratings of physician concern, and less patient and physician social talk.

It is impossible to determine from these studies the degree to which physicians' communication reflects a measure of cultural bias or insensitivity or some spiral of reaction and response to patient bias and expectation of poor treatment. Nevertheless, minority patients' reports of less than optimal relationships are reflected in the talk of their medical visits, particularly in the emotional domains of exchange.

PHYSICIANS' CULTURAL BACKGROUND: INTERNATIONAL MEDICAL GRADUATES

The lack of diversity among U.S. medical students does not mean that the medical workforce lacks ethnic diversity. International medical graduates (IMGs), defined by the Educational Commission for Foreign Medical Graduates (ECFMG) as any physician who has completed basic medical training outside of North America and Puerto Rico (including U.S. citizens), now account for more than 25% of all practicing physicians, and 25% of residents and fellows training in U.S. graduate medical programs (ECFMG 2002 Annual Report, 2002; McMahon, 2004). Although the single largest group of IMGs consists of U.S. citizens, representing a quarter of all IMGs, the great majority of IMG physicians do not share a common ethnicity, culture, or even language with the patients they serve (ECFMG 2002 Annual Report, 2002). Foreign-born IMGs come from a host of countries, with the largest numbers coming from India (21%) and the Philippines (9%), followed by Cuba (4%), Pakistan (4%), and Iran (3.1%) (McMahon, 2004).

The ECFMG has gatekeeper responsibility for IMG entry into U.S. training programs. While the Test of English as a Foreign Language (TOEFL) and the basic and clinical science portions of the U.S. Medical Licensing Examination have been the primary selection criteria for decades, relatively weak performance of IMGs on a variety of competency indices, including clinical skills, has pressured the ECFMG to develop more predictive criteria for IMG selection (Whelan, Gary, Kostis, Boulet, & Hallock, 2002). In response, the ECFMG developed the clinical skills assessment (CSA) exam in 1998 as a measure of clinical, linguistic, and technical readiness for entry into U.S. programs.

The CSA exam is comprised of 10 standardized patient interviews through which student performance is evaluated on several skill dimensions. The measures reflecting interpersonal communication include the standardized patient ratings (from unsatisfactory [1] to excellent [4]) of the following: interviewing and collecting information, counseling and delivering information, rapport, and personal manner. In addition, the standardized patients rate the students' spoken English on a scale from low comprehensibility (1) to very high comprehensibility (4).

Although there has been relatively little research relating the CSA test scores directly to performance with patients, one study examined the question indirectly. Nurses who worked with the IMG residents throughout their clinical rotations were asked to rate the residents' communication skills. The nurses' ratings showed a weak to moderate relationship to the CSA scores (Pearson correlation = 0.39) and spoken English (Pearson correlation = 0.49), suggesting that the test does have some validity in predicting performance (Whelan, McKinley, Boulet, Macrae, & Kamholz, 2001).

Even physicians who pass the variety of ECFMG tests, however, may find themselves unprepared to deal with the great variety of lifestyles, sex-role behaviors, street slang, regional dialects, and biases they are likely to encounter (Cole-Kelly, 1994; Fiscella, Roman-Diaz, Bee-Horng, Botelho, & Frankel, 1997). The cultural adaptation for many IMGs is not limited to the majority U.S. culture. Some two-thirds of IMG physicians work in medically underserved areas, often providing primary care to poor and ethnically diverse patient populations (McMahon, 2004).

These challenges take a toll. In an analysis of anonymous comments by IMG residents on their experiences in caring for patients during residency, Fiscella and colleagues found that fear of rejection and discrimination by U.S. patients was common, as well as concern that language and cultural barriers might interfere with their ability to deliver patient care (Fiscella et al., 1997). For instance, one IMG wrote, "The moment I entered his [the patient's] room and asked him about his problem, he commented on my casual way of dressing. He commented on my not wearing a tie, my footwear, which he thought was highly inappropriate, and my accent which was above all too much for him to accept" (Fiscella et al., 1997, p. 113). Another IMG resident reported a patient saying, "I don't want any doc who can't speak English taking care of me" (Fiscella et al., 1997, p. 113).

Several residents relayed experiences reflecting their frustration at not being able to communicate effectively with their patients—for instance, a resident wrote, "I had difficulty expressing myself on different occasions. Patients and relatives have thought that I have not been caring much. At times, I had difficulty understanding especially the inner city language and I have not been able to take an adequate history" (Fiscella et al., 1997, p. 113). Two male IMGs noted how their cultural background affected their ability to care for female patients, both clinically and emotionally. In the first instance, a resident explained: "Coming from a culture where men do not perform a physical examination of a female patient, it is not easy to do female exam by a male physician, especially breast and genitalia exam" (Fiscella et al., 1997, p. 113). In a second example, the resident wrote "She's supposed to start chemotherapy this morning, and she was crying. We were visiting her and I did not know how to express my support to her, and she's crying. Being from a culture as a female and male there is a difference. You cannot get too close. Things like that. So there was a hesitance. You know, as to how I could hold her, how I could give her comfort" (Fiscella et al., 1997, p. 114).

Considering these special challenges, it is not surprising that IMGs have much higher attrition rates from U.S. residency training programs than do U.S. medical graduates. For instance, the 10-year attrition rate (1981–1991) for IMGs in family practice was 18.5%, more than double the number for U.S. graduates (7.8%) (Laufenburg, Turkal, & Baumgardner, 1994). In a similar vein, IMG physicians report less career satisfaction than U.S. physicians, another likely indicator of cultural strain and practice pressures (Leigh, Kravitz, Schembri, Samuels, & Mobley, 2002).

SOCIAL CLASS

Less attention has been paid to the upper-middle-class profile of medical students than their ethnicity and gender, although these characteristics are related. At current rates (2003–2004), tuition for four years at a state-supported medical school will average $64,000; additional costs for living expenses, books, and equipment, are likely to bring the total cost of a medical education to more than $140,000 (Morrison, 2005). Tuition at a private medical school, like Harvard or Johns Hopkins, is twice as high as a public counterpart, with total costs over four years estimated to exceed $225,000. The high cost of medical education has contributed to a spiraling debt burden. The average medical student owed less than $30,000 at graduation in the 1980s; estimates of debt in 2003 run four times as high (Morrison, 2005).

Considering the economic ramifications of medical training, it is not surprising that some 60% of medical students come from families among the top 20% of income brackets while only 20% of students are from families represented among the lower 60% of income (Jolly, 2004). As parental income increases, there is a consistent increase in the percentage of students who apply to medical school and in the percentage who are accepted. Cooper's analysis of medical school applicants for the years 1982–2002 found that family income, along with parental expectations and education, profoundly influenced the likelihood that a child would apply to medical school (R. A. Cooper, 2003). Family income may also explain the absence of underrepresented minorities in medical school, as Morrison notes that the number one reason given by minority students for not applying to medical school is the cost (Morrison, 2005).

The pathway by which students arrive at a decision to become doctors also appears to reinforce the connection between the middle classes and medicine. Studying about 750 medical students, Rogoff (1957) found that half said they first considered becoming a doctor in their early teens and even younger. An impressive number of these students made their decision to enter medicine so early that the author characterized them as "born with a stethoscope in their ear."

Early decision making is especially common for children of physicians. The sons and daughters of doctors were almost twice as likely as those without a medical parent to have considered medicine as their future career before the teenage years (Rogoff, 1957). The strong evidence of inter-generational links in medicine is related in some measure to the very early socialization of children in medical households to aspire to medical careers, as well as the help, both material and emotional, their families are likely to give them. This is as true now as it was 50 years ago. A recent U.K. study of medical students suggests this effect is still strong; as many as 18% of medical students were the sons or daughters of physicians (Rees & Sheard, 2002).

The importance of the physician's social class background to physician communication and patient care has been addressed—to some extent. Waitzkin analyzed the audiotapes of 34 doctors from varying social class backgrounds in medical visits with some 300 patients (Waitzkin, 1985). Doctors from upper- or upper-middle-class backgrounds compared with those from working-class backgrounds tended to spend more time informing their patients about their conditions, giving more explanations, and providing responses that were at the same technical level as the questions asked. The study concluded: "Orientation to verbal behavior may be a class-linked phenomenon which affects doctors as well as patients. Thus, doctors from working-class backgrounds may differ in their verbal behavior from doctors who come from a higher class position" (Waitzkin, 1985, p. 92).

Also relevant to social class distinctions among physicians are the findings from a large survey of physicians that found that those who rose to the middle class reported greater attitudinal acceptance and behavioral accommodation to consumerist-type challenges than those who originally came from upper- and upper-middle-class backgrounds (Haug & Lavin, 1983). These attitudes may reflect a more dismissive, take-charge orientation of physicians from higher social-class origins compared with a greater appreciation for pragmatic realities of those who are upwardly mobile.

POLITICAL ORIENTATION

Physicians hold political views across the entire political spectrum. Nevertheless, physicians have been long regarded as politically conservative (Mechanic, 1974), as are most medical students (Coe, 1970). A conservative political orientation is not surprising considering the social-class background of most physicians. Like those in other walks of life, "the ideology of physicians depends on background characteristics, the nature of their work, and their self-interest. In general, physicians who tend to support social reform are those who appear to have the least to lose from it" (Mechanic, 1978, p. 399). More recent surveys show little contemporary change in political leanings; a nationwide random survey of physicians in 2001 found that only 17% of respondents label themselves as liberal while most self-identify as politically moderate (49%) or conservative (35%) (Whitney et al., 2001). The AMA leadership is even more politically conservative than its membership. In this same survey, members of the AMA House of Delegates described themselves almost equally as conservative (43%) or moderate (46%), with only 11% self identifying as liberal.

There is a practical consequence of political orientation for the conduct of medical practice. Liberal compared with conservative physicians believe more strongly that the physician should act as a role model for their patients in health habits and play an active role in terms of preventive health counseling with their patients (Maheux, Pineault, & Beland, 1987). Considering that preventive health counseling is both a nonreimbursable and time-consuming task, it is not surprising to note that liberal doctors have lower incomes, see fewer patients per day, and are more likely to believe that they have a responsibility to advise and care for the psychological problems of patients than more conservative physicians (Mechanic, 1974).

Perhaps related to liberal physicians' greater sense of responsibility for the psychological care of patients, political orientation is also related to views regarding medico-social issues such as assisted suicide. Almost half (47%) of liberal physicians in a national survey supported legalization of physician-assisted suicide, compared with 19% of conservative physicians (Whitney et al., 2001). The same survey also found that religious affiliation and intensity of religious belief were powerful predictors of physician attitudes toward assisted suicide. Forty-five percent of Catholic physicians, 32% of Protestant, and 16% of Jewish physicians opposed assisted suicide; moreover, physicians who reported that religion was "very important" to them were far more likely to oppose legislation allowing assisted suicide (55%) than physicians for whom religion was "moderately" (23%) or "not at all" important (18%). Aside from politics and religion, no other physician characteristic, including age, ethnicity, gender, specialty, AMA membership, time spent with the terminally ill, or living in a state with assisted suicide legislation, was related to physician attitudes on this topic.

Political orientation is also associated with practice characteristics (Linn & Lewis, 1979; Mechanic, 1974). Studying a national sample of primary care physicians, Mechanic (1974) found that physicians' political views were highly correlated with the way they viewed the organization and delivery of medical care. Office-based, solo practitioners were more conservative than physicians in groups or in hospital-based practice, while doctors in prepaid practice and academic medicine were most likely to hold liberal political views.

Because of the patient-dependent nature of fee-for-service practice, Mechanic maintained that this form is more personalized and responsive than prepaid group practice. The latter, because of its bureaucratic nature, is said to encourage a more assembly-line, less personal type of practice with physician responsiveness to the organization superseding responsiveness to the patient (Mechanic, 1974). This is especially evident when the bureaucracy's need to cut costs places the physician in a gatekeeper role, controlling access to services and thereby preventing client abuse of the system through over-utilization. Indeed, there are lower rates of surgery, hospitalization, and testing in HMOs than in hospital-based or fee-for-service medical practice (Eisenberg, 1986).

Another characteristic of the prepaid practice is the contractual nature of the arrangement and the conversion of patients into bureaucratic clients. "Clients did not, like customers, threaten to take their business elsewhere; they demanded their rights under their contract and threatened bureaucratic trouble" (Freidson, 1975, p. 52). The threat of recourse to the HMO administrator or other institutional framework gives patients the additional bargaining power of a third party ally with weapons of paperwork and red tape. This potential weapon may afford patients influence even above that held by fee-paying patients seeing doctors in private practice.

An awareness and accommodation to the bureaucratic client may explain the finding that physicians in prepaid practice were more responsive to consumerist-type patient demands than fee-for-service physicians (Haug & Lavin, 1983). Two-thirds of the doctors in prepaid settings reported some form of accommodation to patient demand, in contrast to 15% accommodation by fee-for-service practitioners. Linn and Lewis (1979) similarly reported from their survey that physicians who were employed in a group practice or clinic were more likely to hold favorable attitudes to patient self-care than those engaged in solo medical practice.

Finally, as suggested by the marked differences in attitudes described above, there is some evidence that political orientation affects the doctor-patient dynamic in actual medical encounters. In this regard, Waitzkin (1985) found that more politically liberal doctors tended to give patients more overall explanations and more explanations in understandable language than other doctors.

PROFESSIONAL READINESS FOR A CAREER IN MEDICINE

While gender, ethnicity, and social class describe the sociodemographic profile of physicians, these characteristics do not comprise measures of aptitude or suitability for a career in medicine. The Flexner Report of 1910 is often regarded as a watershed event in enhancing the quality of medical education through the establishment of a scientific curriculum. Perhaps less well known, the report was equally influential in advocating for a systematic method of student selection based on academic qualification. By the 1920s, one in five medical students were leaving school for academic reasons and it was clear that a standardized measure of academic readiness was needed (McGaghie, 2002). In response to these pressures, in 1928 the Association of American Medical Colleges (AAMC) developed the Medical College Admissions Test (MCAT) to systematically assess quantitative and problem solving skills as applied to the biological and physical sciences (McGaghie, 2002). Along with college grades, the MCAT continues to be used by most medical schools as the primary criterion for student selection.

Because of the focus on academic qualification, competition for medical school admission begins during the premed college years. College undergraduates determined to enter medical school show signs and symptoms of what has been termed the "premed syndrome," including "aggressive competitiveness, self-interested pursuit of grades, narrow-minded overspecialization, high anxiety, and more than occasional incidents of academic dishonesty" (Fox, 1989, p. 98). These experiences are not inconsequential in molding and selecting the people who will ultimately become doctors, and they foreshadow the medical school experience.

This is not to suggest that consideration of student readiness for medical training has been limited to the domains of academic preparation, or that the aggressive competitiveness and self-interest described by Fox are indicative of the personal characteristics most valued by medical school interviewers when screening candidates. Professional appreciation for the qualities of personal character that define a good physician, and distinguish a good candidate for medical training, appear throughout the history of medicine. Such traits as compassion, personal integrity, coping capabilities, joint decision-making approaches, respectful and sensitive interprofessional and interpersonal relations, and physical and motivational staying power are often noted in writings in the area (Albanese, Snow, Skochelak, Huggett, & Farrell, 2003; McGaghie, 2002). The problem in using character as an admission criterion to medical school is not in agreement on desirable attributes, although the list is very long, but that the measurement of personal character is so problematic. While many medical schools use the applicant interview, admission essays, and letters of recommendation to ferret out matters of character, few schools claim to have more than weak confidence in their ability to make these assessments in a valid and reliable manner (Albanese et al., 2003).

Even aside from measurement, the stability of these traits may be raised as an issue. Although some investigators have maintained that character solidifies by age 18, Albanese and colleagues disagree (Albanese et al., 2003). The investigators suggest that immersion in the medical school culture does in fact mold student attitudes and values in ways that define a student's professional development. Indeed, indications are that medical students are affected by training and that their attitudes change as they progress through medical school—they become more *negative.*

Most investigators agree that student idealism is high upon entering medical school, although there is no agreement on what happens from then on. It has been suggested that youthful idealism matures to a more reality-based vision of medicine, or is simply suspended during the training period, but that students resume a basic idealism once schooling is complete (Crandall, Volk, & Loemker, 1993; Kurtz & Chalfant, 1991; Light, 1975). No investigators credit the medical training process with inspiring or furthering anything that could be considered even close to idealism or humanism.

In an unusual cohort study of medical students' attitudes toward a variety of social issues in medicine, Woloschuk and colleagues followed three consecutive medical classes (1999–2001) upon entering medical school and as they progressed through their preclinical years to clinical clerkships (Woloschuk, Harasym, & Temple, 2004). Although student attitudes were highly positive at the start of training, there was a substantial decline over time in a variety of areas, including an appreciation for the role of social determinants of patient health, value for the emotional and interpersonal dimensions of the doctor-patient relationship and the role of communication, and regard for cooperation and team building with other health professions. The decline in attitudes toward doctor-patient communication was especially striking at just the time these students began to establish relationships with patients during the clerkship year. Others have similarly noted a decline in positive attitudes toward patients during clerkships, including studies finding that medical students become less patient-centered and more paternalistic in their attitudes (Haidet et al., 2002), less favorably disposed toward to providing care to medically indigent patients (Crandall et al., 1993), less idealistic and less positive in regard to the elderly and patients in chronic pain (Griffith & Wilson, 2001), and less inclined to believe in the importance of discussing psychosocial concerns (G. C. Williams & Deci, 1996).

Why would positive attitudes decline once students begin seeing patients? Some suggest that the emphasis on basic science during the preclinical years is out of proportion with its relevance to clinical practice, and that the critical skills in communicating and relating to patients get short shrift in the medical curriculum. Indeed, in their early years of medical school, students do a better job of talking with their patients than fully trained doctors. As students' medical education progressed, the "science" of medicine replaced its human dimension and students found it harder simply to talk with patients. What were enjoyable talks with patients during the first years became awkward hypothesis-testing sessions in later years with an accelerated decline in communication skills during the fourth year of training (Helfer, 1970). It appears that as training progresses, students appeared to "miss the forest for the trees" and lose their grasp on the patient's total health picture by their single-minded focus on biomedical issues (Martin, Gilson, Bergner, Bobbitt, Pollard, Conn, & Cole, 1976).

More recent studies suggest that little has changed in the 20-odd years since the above studies were conducted. The decline in interpersonal communication skills and positive attitudes toward patients, particularly during 4th year clerkships, has continued (Pfeiffer, Madray, Ardolino, & Willms, 1998; Griffith, Haist, Wilson, & Rich, 1996; Griffith, Rich, & Wilson, 1995). The pattern of skill decline is particularly evident in the work of Pfeiffer and colleagues. These investigators tracked the communication skills of three cohorts of medical students for four years using standardized patient ratings of their performance in at least one interview each year. The pattern of findings was virtually the same for all three cohorts. Social history-taking skills showed small increases over the first two years but a substantial decline in years three and four, while communication skills and rapport-building skills showed increases to year three and then a decline in year four. The authors concluded that the gains evident in the first two or three years were overshadowed by pressures of patient care during clerkships. This pressure is made worse by exposure to residents and attending physicians serving as role models for medical students who are themselves preoccupied with the challenges of differential diagnosis and the elimination of any activity that may be considered superfluous, such as the psychosocial dimensions of care and skillful communication with patients (Pfeiffer et al., 1998).

While the formal curriculum is well annotated in school catalogues, Hafferty suggests that it is the hidden or informal curriculum that conveys the seminal lessons in the development of professional identity (Hafferty, 1998). The actions of harried role models observed with patients and colleagues under pressure appear to have a far more lasting impression on students and their conceptions of professionalism than all the hours spent in the classroom. The work of the informal curriculum becomes evident during clerkships and accelerates through internship, residency, and fellowship training.

The negative effects of distancing physicians from patients is accentuated in the hospital training experience in what has been characterized as an especially alienating and punishing way (Klass, 1987; Mizrahi, 1986). Despite the privileged backgrounds of most medical students, the hospital training experience is one of deprivation. The trainees are continually tested, both physically and emotionally, to prove their dedication to medicine with constant sleep deprivation and highly stressful work conditions (Butterfield, 1988; Daugherty, Baldwin, & Rowley, 1998).

A rare window into the nature of residency training was provided by sociologist Terry Mizrahi (1986) in her systematic, 3-year observational study of the lives of interns and residents at a large university medical center. Mizrahi concluded that the most important lesson learned during the early months of training, and one that was reinforced throughout the trainee's career, was how to "GROP" (get rid of patients)—that is, discharge one's responsibility for patients as quickly as possible. "GROP became an art form within the house staff subculture, and those who were especially good at it were esteemed and called 'dispo kings'" (p. 166). Patients were seen as but one more obstacle to seeing their family or getting some sleep (Mizrahi, 1986). Mizrahi concluded that "the educational experience is structured to militate against the development of humanistic doctor-patient relationships . . . the novices are systematically dehumanized, which only fosters the deterioration of the doctor-patient relationship rather than allowing it to develop as something positive" (p. 119).

All aspects of deprivation—psychological as well as physical—endured by interns and residents acted to extinguish any initial idealism and concern for patients the student may have had. Moreover, Mizrahi suggested that the frustrations experienced by the young doctors while in training were taken out on patients. In her words, it was a case of "one category of victims—albeit, temporary ones—victimizing a second weaker category" (Mizrahi, 1986, p. 166).

There were some exceptions to the GROP rule. Some patients were valued; patients who presented complex symptoms or a form of rare disease that may be used by the attending faculty and house staff for "clinical material" or teaching purposes were sought after. Further, it was noted that in addition to how interesting their case was, patients were classified on another continuum reflecting care burden and ranging from ideal to despised. The ideal patient was "middle class, intelligent without questioning the doctor's judgment, clean, deferential, helpful, cooperative, and so forth. The despised patient was one defined in the subculture as an abuser: a self-abuser, system abuser, house staff abuser or some combination" (Mizrahi, 1986, p. 167). The extent of derision and bad feelings toward despised patients was reflected in a vocabulary of insults directed toward patients. "GOMERs" (patients they wanted to "get out of my emergency room"), trainwrecks (patients with serious multiple medical problems), scumbags, dirtbags, crocks, garbage, junk, and "SHPOs" (subhuman pieces of shit) were terms repeatedly used to characterize patients, at times within earshot of the patient (Mizrahi, 1986). Any sympathy at all for patients was suppressed by the increasingly technical or procedural orientation toward patients, screening out any more subtle or subjective considerations. In this process, psychosocial and environmental factors were for the most part simply ignored, or under the best of circumstances deferred to other health professionals, most commonly social workers.

Several of the physicians observed throughout their training in the Mizrahi study were interviewed five and six years later (Mizrahi, 1986). The doctors in the follow-up were found to have softened their views of patients to some extent. Particularly those physicians who went into private practice, as opposed to academic medicine, had redefined their notion of optimal health care by decreasing the importance of technical and academic expertise and increasing the importance of considering the "whole" patient (Mizrahi, 1986).

While new rules put into effect in 2003 by the Accreditation Council for Graduate Medical Education (ACGME) have substantially reduced the total number of hours residents may work per week and limited the number of continuous duty hours, residents can still be required to work 80 hour weeks and up to 30 hours without a break (Philibert, Friedmann, & Williams, 2005). The concerns that prompted implementation of these rules, that over-worked and sleep-deprived residents may be prone to make serious and sometimes deadly mistakes, have been alleviated by the new rules, but not entirely dismissed (Asch & Parker, 1988; Veasey, Rosen, Barzansky, Rosen, & Owens, 2002). Nevertheless, there is evidence that the work hour restric-tion has achieved at least some of its desired effect. Not only do residents report a substantial decline in their on call and work schedules, but these changes have also has a positive affect on role modeling to the medical stu-dents they supervise. A survey of medical students completing required clinical rotations before and after the hour restrictions were implemented found that their ratings of their primary resident's availability and interest improved and that fewer students reported choosing their specialty or con-sidering leaving medicine based on concerns about lifestyle and long hours (Jagsi, Shapiro, & Weinstein, 2005).

PHYSICIAN PERSONALITY TRAITS

We know that some medical specialties attract particular kinds of personal-ities and values. Indeed, generalizations regarding specialty-types are so well entrenched in medical lore that doctor stereotypes are among the best known of the doctor jokes. Take, for example, the Duck Joke, described by Sharon Farber in her humor website as the classical doctor joke with infinite varia-tions (http://jophan.org/mimosa/m29/farber.htm):

A general practitioner, an internist, and a surgeon go duck hunting. A duck flies overhead, and the internist sights it and says, "By the wing span and the way it flaps its wings and its plumage, I'd say it is almost certain to be a pheasant. But I couldn't exclude it being a grouse." No shot was taken. Another duck flies overhead, and the GP sights it and says, "Gee, kinda looks like a duck," and shoots it. A third bird flies overhead. The surgeon raises his gun and shoots. Then he looks at the others. "What was that?" he asks.

The Duck Joke characterization resonates with that of the social psychology literature. As noted by David Mechanic, "The image of the internist is that of the intellectual problem solver, while the surgeon is seen as more aggressive and active. The family practitioner, in contrast, tends to be less conceptual and more gregarious than the internist (Mechanic, 1978, p. 382). The primary source for this type of personality characterization is the Myers-Briggs Type Inventory (MBTI), a widely used measure of personality that has been used in studies of medical students and physicians since its development in the 1950s (Stilwell, Wallick, Thal, & Burleson, 2000). Based on Jung's theory of personality, the inventory assesses an individual's proclivity for particular ways of seeing and solving problems. Variation is scored along a four-dimensional continuum: perceiving (sensing-intuition), with sensing types perceiving the immediate facts of their experiences while intuitive types focus on possibilities and meanings; deciding (thinking—feeling), with thinking types making decisions impersonally and objectively while feeling types make more subjective and personal decisions; orientation (extraversion—introversion), with extraverts tending toward actions and objects while introverts tend toward concepts and ideas; and, coping (judging—perception), with judging types tending toward a planned and orderly manner while perceiving types are more spontaneous and flexible (Ornstein, Markert, Johnson, Rust, & Afrin, 1988).

One way in which the MBTI has been used with medical students is in the prediction of medical specialization. Although there had been no large-scale studies of medical students since the late 1970s, Stilwell and colleagues found that many individual medical schools had continued to use the measure with their students, usually administering the test during the student's first year (Stilwell et al., 2000). The investigators were successful in gaining access to MBTI measures from 12 U.S. medical schools with data on almost 4,000 students who had graduated between 1983 and 1995. These measures were then related to specialty choice, based on information provided through the National Residency Matching Program, Military Match, or the Early Specialty Match. The MBTI types were clearly related to specialty choice. The factors strongly predictive of choosing a career in primary care were being introverted and feeling types; even among this group, the highest feeling types chose family medicine over other primary care areas. The people-oriented nature of primary care with its rewards coming from long-term relationships with families, rather than such things as money and prestige, provides some explanation for its appeal to students scoring high on the feeling and introversion dimension. Among the graduates who chose nonprimary care, the analysis found that those choosing surgical specialties were more likely to be extroverted thinker types. In this instance, surgeons' proclivity for objective and impersonal action fits the demands of surgical work and its need to

be decisive and unemotional. Further, the status and monetary rewards of surgical specialties are especially appealing to extroverts (Stilwell et al., 2000).

Gender was important in career selection as well, with disproportionate
representation of females in primary care and males in surgical specialties
(Stilwell et al., 2000). There are a host of reasons for gender preferences,
some of which are discussed in Chapter 6; however, gender was independent
of the MBTI prototypes, with both male and female introverts and feelers
choosing primary care while male and female extraverts and thinking types
chose surgical specialties.

The MBTI has also been related to test-ordering behaviors of physicians.
Test ordering is a particular area of interest, not only because of the costs
involved, but also because it reflects differential attitudes towards technology
and uncertainty—both issues with implications for the way the doctor is
likely to communicate with patients. Based on a study of 53 family medicine
physicians monitored over a three-year period, the MBTI personality variables introversion/extroversion and sensing/intuition were more significant
predictors of whether the physician ordered a test than any of the other
aspects studied, including a variety of patient sociodemographic, utilization,
and physical status variables. Introverted and intuitive physicians were found
to order more laboratory tests for their hypertensive patients than did their
more extroverted and sensing colleagues (Ornstein et al., 1988). By way of
explanation, the authors suggest that physicians with tendencies toward both
introversion and intuition are likely to consider the many subtleties and uncer-
tainties in a course of action and so seek additional objective information
through tests before deciding upon a treatment. Extroverts and sensing types,
in contrast, are more likely to trust their perceptions and go forward with a
treatment plan in a more direct and aggressive manner without the need to
validate their perceptions with tests.

The implications of these personality types for patterns of communication
with patients are many. One might speculate that in relying heavily on tests
for decision-making data, introverted and intuitive physicians are more prone
to ignore the potential diagnostic clues their patients may offer. In these cases
high test use may be in lieu of talking with patients, preferring the more
"objective" information of tests to the sometimes confusing thread of a
patient's story of his or her illness.

An intriguing question is whether attitudinal attributes such as those
reflected in the MBTI are further reinforced by the medical school the student
attends. For instance, Epstein and colleagues found that students from medical schools with a research orientation ordered far more tests than students in
practice-focused schools (Epstein, Begg, & McNeil, 1984). The authors note
that while it is possible that trainees with a predisposition to use technical services self-select into particular types of schools and training programs, it is

also true that the environments of these schools shape the development of clinical habits, and perhaps reinforce attitudinal predispositions oriented toward high use of diagnostic tests (Epstein et al., 1984).

It is noteworthy that regardless of the links that may have been made between MBTI scores and any particular physician practice, from the very earliest studies of MBTI types investigators have concluded that the tasks of medicine are so diverse that it appeals to, and gains strength from, students of all psychological types (Stilwell et al., 2000).

PHYSICIAN ATTITUDES TOWARD PATIENT CARE

As noted in previous chapters, the practice of patient-centered medicine requires an appreciation for the broad life context of the patient and the ability to incorporate both psychological and biomedical aspects into patient care. Physicians vary, however, in the extent to which they believe that their medical responsibility extends to patients' psychological and emotional problems. A measure of physician attitudes toward the psychosocial aspects of patient care, the Physician Belief Scale (PBS), was developed by Ashworth and colleagues to quantify individual physician variation along these lines and to compare the attitudes of physicians across primary care specialties (Ashworth, Williamson, & Montano, 1984). Example items (5-point scale ranging from strongly disagree to strongly agree) are: "Consideration of psychosocial problems will require more effort than I have to give," "I do not focus on psychosocial problems until I have ruled out organic disease," and "I am intruding when I ask psychosocial questions."

Based on administration of the scale to a convenience sample of 91 primary care physicians and eight psychiatrists, the authors not only found substantial variation among physicians in PBS scores, but also significant differences across specialties. As one might expect, psychiatrists had the strongest PBS scores. Internists had significantly weaker PBS scores than both psychiatrists and family physicians, and pediatricians scored midway between family physicians and internists (Ashworth et al., 1984).

If physicians vary so much on the PBS, treatment of patients may vary as well. For instance, a physician who considers a patient's job stress and family discord when attempting to understand why the patient's hypertension remains uncontrolled is more likely to discuss these matters with the patient and consider recommendations that include stress reduction and marital counseling in addition to drug management. Physician scores on the PBS were related to visit communication in a study evaluating the effect of two communication skills programs on doctor-patient communication (Levinson & Roter, 1995). Physician scores were comparable to the earlier study, with internists scoring substantially weaker than family practice physicians. Among the 50 physicians studied, those with stronger psychosocial attitudes engaged in more explicitly emotional exchanges with their patients and used fewer closed-ended questions during their visits. These physicians were also judged to be more interested, dominant, and responsive by coders, suggesting greater animation and involvement in the interaction. Not only were physician attitudes related to physician communication, but patients of these physicians also used a distinct pattern of communication: they offered more psychosocial (and less biomedical) information to their physicians, were more emotionally expressive (i.e., expressed feelings, showed concern, and asked for reassurance) and were more engaged in the dialogue both verbally and nonverbally.

Several other attitude measures have also been used to explore physicians' psychosocial and patient-centered orientation to patient care and specialty choice. For instance, Dutch researchers have used the Doctor-Patient Scale as a measure of patient-centeredness. The 48-item, five-point scale includes items like "Listening to patients is more efficient than talking to them" and "Clinical competence is based on knowledge and skills, very little on attitude" (Batenburg, Smal, Lodder, & Melker, 1999). Based on surveys of Dutch medical students and postgraduate trainees, the investigators found that patient centeredness scores were related to intended and actual specialty choice but unrelated to level of training or gender. Students anticipating a career in surgery and surgical trainees both showed lower patient-centered attitudes than primary care trainees or students in primary care clerkships.

Krupat and colleagues in the U.S. developed the Patient-Practitioner Orientation Scale (PPOS) in a somewhat similar way to reflect the patient-centeredness of medical students and physicians (Krupat, Hiam, Fleming, & Freeman, 1999). The 18-item scale includes items like "The most important part of the standard medical visit is the physical exam" and "If doctors are truly good at diagnosis and treatment, the way they relate to patients is not that important." The investigators found that PPOS scores were highest among female medical students, students interested in community and primary care practice, and students with positive attitudes toward psychosocial issues.

Increasing recognition of the importance of physician attitudes for patient care is likely to spur more work in this area. Further discussion of physician attitudes in relation to the outcomes of care, both patient and physician, is presented in Chapter 9, as we consider the consequences of doctor-patient communication.

6

The Influence of Physician Gender on Communication: Why Physician Gender (Especially) Matters in Communication

More than any other physician sociodemographic characteristic, gender does matter, at least in relation to communication and the doctor-patient relationship. We will approach the topic from several directions. First we will discuss the increasing presence of women in the medical workforce and the implications of a gender shift on medical specialization and work life, including the growing trend toward part-time medical practice. These factors are important in understanding the context in which female physicians practice medicine.

Next, we will describe how gender affects visit communication. In this regard, we will review the results of two meta-analytic reviews of physician gender and communication that we have conducted over the past few years. The first of these relates physician gender to their own communication during medical encounters, addressing the question of how, and to what extent, do male and female doctors differ in their communication with patients (Roter, Hall, & Aoki, 2002). One might argue that the focus on physician communication fails to appreciate the influence of patients in shaping the doctor-patient relationship. In fact, discussions of gender effects in medical communication have virtually ignored the question of how patients behave toward male versus female physicians. This is an important question, however, because it shifts a largely physician-centric view of communication to one that better appreciates the reciprocal and dynamic elements of both patient and physician in the medical interchange. Therefore, the results of our second meta-analytic review on how, and to what extent, patients differ in their communication toward male and female doctors will also be presented (J. A. Hall & Roter, 2002).

THE INCREASING PRESENCE OF WOMEN IN THE MEDICAL WORKFORCE

The sociodemographic profile that has traditionally characterized the medical profession as disproportionately male is changing. The most dramatic change has been in the spectacular increases in the percentage of women entering medical school. The trends evident even in the 1970s and 1980s during which there was a seven-fold increase, from 5 to 37%, in enrollment of women in the 1960s compared with the 1980s (Jonas & Etzel, 1988), continued to skyrocket throughout the 1990s. Female applicants to medical school outnumbered males (by about 1%) for the first time in the 2003–2004 academic year and only slightly fewer than half (49.7%) of the entering class of more than 16,500 medical students in 2004 was female. Furthermore, women are predicted to comprise 57% of the medical school applicant pool by 2020 (R. A. Cooper, 2003). The growing inclusion of women in the medical workforce is not only an American phenomenon. The proportion of all medical students who are female has also grown in Europe. A recent review notes that more than half of current medical students in the Netherlands, the U.K., and Australia are women (Heiligers & Hingstman, 2000). In Eastern Europe and in Israel, women have long dominated the medical workforce (Harden, 2001).

It is notable that women are expected to account for the entire growth in the number of medical applicants in the U.S. over the next two decades. Moreover, women are likely to replace both Caucasian male medical students, as well as male medical students of color. By 2020, women will represent 55% of Caucasian and Asian applicants, 60% of Hispanic applicants, and almost 70% African American medical school applicants (R. A. Cooper, 2003). Consequently, it appears that male minority physicians will constitute the growing under-represented sociodemographic group in medicine in the next 15 years.

PHYSICIAN GENDER AND MEDICAL SPECIALIZATION

The distribution of female physicians across specialties is not random. Female physicians have traditionally chosen, and continue to choose, primary care specialties; they are disproportionately represented in pediatrics, internal medicine, family practice, and especially, obstetrics-gynecology. For the most part, these specialties carry the greatest lifestyle burden in terms of uncontrollable work hours and are the lowest paid of the medical professions (Dorsey, Jarjoura, & Rutecki, 2005). In commenting on the nature of gender-related specialization, Levinson and Lurie (2004) note that female physicians are more likely to undertake roles that are arduous, altruistic, and lacking prestige. Indeed, the authors describe female physicians "as the housewives of the profession, that is, those who take responsibility for the profession's grunt work in their careers as general internists" (p. 472).

While a number of personality characteristics have been linked to specialty preference (see Chapter 5 for a discussion of some of these), Stratton and colleagues suggest that exposure to gender discrimination and sexual harassment in medical school also affects specialty choice (Stratton, McLaughlin, Witte, Fosson, & Nora, 2005). In their study, 10% of male and 27% of female medical students reported personally experiencing gender discrimination and sexual harassment during their selection of a residency program. For these students, 45% of the females and 16% of the males indicated that this experience influenced their choice of medical specialty to some degree.

Women experienced higher levels of discrimination and sexual harassment than males in every specialty, with only one exception. In obstetrics and gynecology, male students report more discrimination than their female counterparts (56% versus 38%); moreover, it is in this quarter that discrimination appears to have its greatest effect on career selection. Although fewer men are affected by gender discrimination than women, men have reported that these experiences affected their specialty and residency program decisions to a greater degree than it affected women (Stratton et al., 2005). It is noteworthy that the number of men entering obstetrics and gynecology has declined dramatically over the past 15 years—from 6.4% in 1990 to 2% in 2003, raising the possibility that there will be no men entering the profession by the end of the decade.

The number of female physicians choosing obstetrics and gynecology also dropped during this time period, from 13.7% to 10.5%, but this decline is less dramatic and consistent with the general trend away from "non-controllable lifestyle" specialties (Dorsey et al., 2005).

Physician Gender and Part-Time Work

Increasing numbers of female physicians in medical school does not directly translate into numbers of practicing female physicians, and, as noted by Mechanic, McAlpine, and Rosenthal (2001), it will be some time before there is equal patient access to physicians of both genders. While the proportion of physicians in office-based practice who are women increased from approximately 13% in 1989 to 20.5% in 1998, the average number of weekly office visits for a male physician is about 35% greater than the average number of visits for female physicians (Mechanic et al., 2001). At least some of this difference is due to increasing numbers of women physicians working part-time or on a reduced schedule. For instance, Cull and colleagues found that female pediatric residents were almost five times as likely to accept part-time positions as their male colleagues (14% versus 3%) and that the female residents anticipated far greater interest in arranging a part-time position within the next 5 years than their male colleagues (58% versus 15%) (Cull et al., 2002). As would be expected, the great majority of women, 93%, reported that they would devote their extra time to meeting family needs related to children.

An interesting perspective on part-time work is provided by Dr. Audrey Shafer (2004), an academic anesthesiologist. Dr. Shafer notes that cutting her work obligation by 50% means that she routinely devotes 35–40 hours per week to patient care. This is not atypical; a recent analysis of physician work hours found that part-time physicians average 32 hours per week, with some working as many as 60 hours per week (physicians in full-time practice average a 49-hour work week, with some working as many as 90 hours per week) (Carr, Gareis, & Barnett, 2003). Both male and female physicians are moving away from the "uncontrollable lifestyle" specialties that make such great demands on time, including primary care and obstetrics-gynecology; however, women are doing so at a lower rate than men (Dorsey et al., 2005).

DO MALE AND FEMALE PHYSICIANS COMMUNICATE DIFFERENTLY?

The issues discussed above, including specialty selection and work hours relate directly to the kind of medicine male and female physicians practice, as well as how they practice medicine and communicate with their patients. In Chapter 4 we summarized some of the differences that have been documented in the interpersonal style of women and men in routine interaction. Women disclose more information about themselves in conversation (Dindia & Allen, 1992), they have a warmer and more engaged style of nonverbal communication and they encourage and facilitate others to talk to them more freely and in a warmer and more intimate way (J. A. Hall, 1984). In contrast to men's tendency to assert status differences, there is evidence that women take greater pains to downplay their own status in an attempt to equalize status with a partner (Eagly & Johnson, 1990). Women have also been shown to be more accurate in judging others' feelings expressed through nonverbal cues and in judging others' personality traits, as well as more accurate in communicating emotion via nonverbal cues (J. A. Hall, 1984).

Our review of the literature found 23 studies that examined physician gender and medical communication (as assessed using neutral observers, audiotapes, or videotapes) published in English between 1967 and 2001. Not all of these studies were of practicing physicians with patients. We included a study if it involved physicians at any level, including physicians in training (interns or residents), or medical students. We also found that as many as one-third of the studies reporting communication findings involved standardized patients, so we included these as well as studies of actual patients.

Once the studies were identified, we abstracted the findings (quantitatively, as appropriate for meta-analysis) and characterized the communication measures and variables that were used.

The first question we address is whether male and female physicians differ in how much time they spend with patients. The answer is yes. With only one exception (one of our own studies of U.S. obstetricians; Roter, Geller, Bernhardt, Larson, & Doksum, 1999), all of the studies that directly measured length of visit in our review found that female physicians conduct longer visits than male physicians. While the average length of visit for male doctors averaged 21 minutes, ranging from 7.5 to 37 minutes, female physicians' visits were 2 minutes longer, averaging 23 minutes and ranging from 10.5 minutes to 37 minutes. The differences in time spent with patients, then, appear greater at the lower, rather than the upper, end of the time range; patients are less likely to have a visit that lasts less than 10 minutes when they are with a female doctor than when they are with a male doctor.

Similar conclusions regarding physician gender and visit length have also been drawn from physician reports. Based on a 10-year analysis (1989 to 1998) of the National Ambulatory Medical Care Survey (NAMCS) of the National Center for Health Statistics (in which the number of sampled visits ranged from 24,715 to 43,469 each year), Mechanic et al. (2001) concluded that patient visits with female physicians, across all specialties, are about 1.2 minutes longer, on average, than visits with male physicians.

Do one or two minutes really make much of a difference? Again, the answer is yes. With increasing time and productivity pressures that plague all physicians, any increase can represent a substantial time burden. And, even small differences in visit length could put a female physician an hour or more behind her male colleagues at the end of a busy day. A report by Bensing and colleagues on gender differences in the practice style of Dutch general practitioners adds an additional surprising insight into the issue of visit length (Bensing, van den Brink-Muinen, & de Bakker, 1993). The researchers reported not only that female Dutch practitioners spent more time with their patients than did their male colleagues, but also that these differences were even more pronounced when the visit length of part-time physicians was examined. Among full-time physicians, 32.7% of visits with female physicians were longer than 10 minutes while 25.7% of male physician visits were this long; for part-time physicians, 34% of female visits and 23.2% of male visits were longer than 10 minutes. (Note: the average length of a consultation in the Netherlands is 8.1 minutes.)

As far as we know, this type of analysis has not been done elsewhere, but we can speculate that the reduced hours of part-time work may act as a safety valve of sorts for female physicians by reducing the pressures of continuously falling behind schedule on a daily basis.

The next question is, how is the time spent? Do female physicians do a bit more of everything, or are there specific areas of communication that receive extra attention? Using a functional model of the medical interview that includes four primary visit tasks, (1) data gathering and facilitation of patient disclosure, (2) patient education and counseling, (3) emotional responsiveness, and (4) partnership building, we found that gender-linked differences were evident in every category. (More detail regarding the four functions of the medical interview and the specific communication elements included in each is provided in Chapter 7.)

In regard to the first of the functions, data gathering, it is evident that female physicians ask more questions of their patients than male physicians. This is very evident in the greater number of psychosocial questions asked, but no conclusions regarding gender effects could be drawn in regard to questions dealing with biomedical topics. There were differences in the format of the questions asked, as well. Female physicians ask more closed-ended questions than their male counterparts; there is no evidence of a gender effect for open-ended questions.

Evidence of gender differences in regard to patient education and counseling, the second function of the medical visit, is mixed. This category is characterized in terms of content, with a focus on either biomedical topics (e.g., medical symptoms and history, diagnosis, prognosis, and treatment) or psychosocial topics (e.g., prevention; lifestyle; quality of life and adjustment; social, family, and work relationships; and issues related to discussions of feelings and emotions). There is little evidence that physician gender affected medically specific counseling, however, as in question asking, there is strong evidence that female physicians engage in more psychosocial discussion with patients than do male physicians.

The third medical function, partnership building, occurs when the physician actively facilitates patient participation in the medical visit and/or attempts to equalize status by assuming a less dominating stance within the relationship. There is no doubt that female physicians more actively facilitate patient participation in the visit than male physicians. The result was somewhat different for the status-equalizing aspect of partnership building, and no clear picture of a gender effect emerged.

Finally, the fourth function, emotional responsiveness, includes explicit inquiry about feelings and emotions, exploration of emotional concerns, and statements of empathy and concern. This category is distinguished from psychosocial exchange by directly expressing feelings and emotions. Female physicians clearly engage in more emotional talk than their male counterparts. Other categories of communication with socioemotional content include positive and negative talk, and social chitchat. Positive talk captures the generally positive atmosphere created in the visit through verbal behaviors such as agreements, encouragement, and reassurance. Several studies also coded positive nonverbal behavior in some manner, for instance smiling and head nods.

No studies reported higher levels of positive talk or positive nonverbal behavior for male physicians, supporting a strong general finding that female physicians were more positive, both verbally and nonverbally, in their communication than male physicians. In contrast, there were no significant gender differences in physicians' use of negative talk or social chitchat.

All in all, the picture suggests somewhat more warmth, responsiveness, and empathy in the medical communication of female than male doctors. This fits with the impressions of medical students, medical school faculty, and directors of medical residency programs that female doctors are less egotistical and more humanistic, sensitive, and altruistic than their male counterparts (Levinson & Lurie, 2004). It is also consistent with research that measures medical students' attitudes about patient care. G. C. Williams and Deci (1996) found that female medical students endorsed the value of discussing psychosocial concerns in medical visits more than male medical students and that they also held a philosophy of patient care that was more autonomy promoting. Indications that female physicians are more patient-centered (from both the observational and the self-report studies) are also consistent with two studies that found that female doctors report liking their patients more than male doctors do when asked about their patients by name (J. A. Hall, Epstein, DeCiantis, & McNeil, 1993; J. A. Hall, Horgan, Stein, & Roter, 2002).

DO PATIENTS COMMUNICATE DIFFERENTLY WITH MALE AND FEMALE DOCTORS?

Behavioral differences in the communication styles of male and female physicians would be especially important if they produce corresponding gender differences in patients' behavior directed back at them. Indeed, the effect of physician gender on patient communication is evident in the small number of studies in which this is measured and these results suggest that patient behavior largely reciprocates gender-linked physician behaviors. Thus, many of the gender differences in physician communication are also evident in the communication of the patients toward male and female physicians.

As was discussed earlier, female physicians have longer visits than males. In analyzing patient talk, we found consistent evidence that at least some of this additional time is taken by patients; patients talk more when with female physicians than they do with male physicians. Why this may be so is suggested through a reciprocal pattern of communication influence.

Patients reciprocated some physician communication behaviors directly and others in a more indirect manner. Direct reciprocation by patients of physician gender-linked communication was evident in more patient facilitation of physician input by asking if they are being understood, paraphrasing what the physician said, and offering interpretations, and being verbally attentive (a constellation of behaviors that we call partnership building) when with female physicians. And, it appears that this aspect of communication mirrors the gender finding for female physicians' communication. Thus, in general medical practice, patients (both male and female) were more inclined toward a partnership relationship with a female physician rather than a male physician. Similarly, patient communication was parallel to those of physicians for positive comments. Positive talk, which included statements of agreement and approval, was more directed toward female physicians, paralleling the physician gender effect for higher levels of female physicians' positive talk.

Indirect reciprocation was evident in patients' information exchange. Even though male and female physicians did not differ in how much biomedical information they provided to their patients, patients of female physicians provided more biomedical information to them than to male physicians. Since female physicians ask more psychosocial questions than their male counterparts, it may be that this type of questioning stimulates more patient disclosure of both a psychosocial and biomedical nature. Higher levels of patient disclosure may also be fostered by female physicians' more active efforts to build partnerships through inviting the patients' opinions and through the use of interest cues, such as uh-huh and nodding, as mentioned above. Interestingly, though female physicians made more emotionally focused statements than male physicians, patients did not direct more emotional statements back to them. Patients did, however, disclose more psychosocial information to their female physicians.

In addition to offering quantitative evidence of patient behavior in the form of frequency counts of different categories of communication, several studies also looked at patients' global (including nonverbal) communication, assessed most often through global ratings of their communication made by neutral observers. There was little evidence that patients displayed more positive global affect to female physicians; however, ratings of patients' assertiveness support a general conclusion that patients were more self-assertive with female than male physicians.

GENDER CONCORDANCE BETWEEN PATIENT AND PHYSICIAN

There have been relatively few studies directly examining the effect of patient and physician gender simultaneously on medical communication, but evidence suggests that same-gender dyads strengthen the communication effects observed in the earlier mentioned reviews. This is consistent with similar effects in nonclinical studies. For example, because women gaze more at others than men do, and in addition people gaze more at women than at men, same-gender pairings show the most extreme differences (J. A. Hall, 1984). Two U.S. studies (J. A. Hall, Irish, Roter, Ehrlich, & Miller, 1994a; Roter, Lipkin, & Korsgaard, 1991) found that visits were longer when both the doctor and patient were female and that there was a more equal contribution of patient and physician to the medical dialogue, compared to visits with other gender combinations. J. A. Hall et al. (1994a) also reported more positive statements, head nodding, and interest cues in female concordant visits compared with other gender combinations.

A large study of medical communication in six Western European countries also found that female concordant dyads were more likely to have longer visits, higher levels of psychosocial discussion, emotional exchange, eye contact, and lower levels of physician verbal dominance (van den Brink-Muinen, van Dulmen, Messerli-Rohrbach, & Bensing, 2002). Notably, the investigators found few country-specific differences in the pattern of results, suggesting that the observed effects of physician and patient gender on communication appear to transcend national and cultural borders.

Despite these communication benefits, at least for female patients in choosing a female physician, most studies reveal only a weak preference for physicians of the same gender when the presenting complaint is not gender-specific (Bensing, van den Brink-Muinen, & de Bakker, 1993; Elstad, 1994; Pearse, 1994; Weisman & Teitelbaum, 1989). Moreover, while female patients are more likely to choose female physicians than male patients, both male and female patients overwhelmingly choose male physicians (Schmittdiel, Grumback, Selby, & Quesenberry, 2000). A preference for a same-gender physician, however, is much stronger when patients are seeking help for intimate health problems, including gynecological and obstetrical care (Elstad, 1994; Pearse, 1994; Weisman & Teitelbaum, 1989). These preferences have been linked to an expectation of special insight and experience with gender-specific problems and embarrassment and discomfort associated with physical exposure and discussion of sensitive matters across gender lines. Perhaps related to some aspect of comfort in the discussion of gender-specific problems, female physicians have been reported to provide more gender-linked preventive services, such as mammograms and pap smears, to their female patients (Bertakis, Helms, Callahan, Azari, & Robbins, 1995; Bensing et al., 1993; J. A. Hall, Palmer, et al., 1990; Henderson & Weisman, 2001; Lurie, Margolis, McGovern, Mink, & Slater, 1997; Schmittdiel et al., 2000; Stafford et al., 1999), as well as more general preventive counseling and mental health counseling for patients of both genders (Bensing et al., 1993; Maheux, Dufort, Beland, Jacques, & Levesque, 1990).

GENDER-LINKED EXPECTATIONS AND JUDGMENTS OF PHYSICIAN BEHAVIOR

The communication behaviors associated with female physicians are those generally valued by patients and predictive of positive patient outcomes. (A detailed discussion of the consequences of communication for patient outcomes will be presented in Chapter 10.) Nevertheless, the literature directly relating physician gender and patient satisfaction is mixed, with some studies finding higher satisfaction with female physicians (Bernzweig, Takayama, Phibbs, Lewis, & Pantell, 1997; C. C. Lewis, Scott, Pantell, & Wolf, 1986; Roter et al., 1999) and others finding the opposite or no effect (J. A. Hall, Irish, Roter, Ehrlich, & Miller, 1994b; Handler, Rosenberg, Raube, & Kelley, 1998; C. E. Ross, Mirowsky, & Duff, 1982). In our own studies, we have also reported mixed results. Based on analysis of two independent studies, we found that both male and female patients of young female physicians reported lower ratings of satisfaction than other patients (J. A. Hall et al., 1994b). An intriguing element of our finding, based on audiotape analysis, was that the communication behaviors generally valued by patients were not associated with patient satisfaction when performed by the young female doctors. We speculate that other patient values and prejudices, perhaps an inferred lack of authority or expertise because of her youth and gender, may offset whatever advantage the young female physician might have by virtue of her communication performance. Alternatively, expectations for positive communication skills (including partnership and emotional support) may have been so high that patients were disappointed despite the performance of these behaviors by their female physicians.

A related interpretation regarding raised expectations for female physicians may be given to the findings of Schmittdiel et al. (2000), who investigated gender preferences and satisfaction in a large managed care organization. Female patients who chose a female physician differed from the small number of male patients who also chose a female physician, and both male and female patients who did not opt to chose a physician at all, in two ways; the female patients who chose a female physician placed a higher value on their physicians' communication skills, and they were less satisfied with the medical care they received from their physicians. In contrast, patients who did not express a gender preference for a physician did not differ in the satisfaction ratings they gave to their physicians in relation to their own gender or the gender of their physician. The significance of these findings may be in the female patients' raised expectations in regard to the interpersonal communication performance of their female physicians. As noted earlier, female physicians engage in more of the communication behaviors generally valued by patients. Nevertheless, even good performance may not be sufficient to meet the high expectations of female patients for their female doctors, particularly under tight scheduling constraints typical of managed care.

A similarly unfair judgment process for male physicians in obstetrics and gynecology may also be evident. Within the context of our own study of male and female obstetricians (Roter et al., 1999) it appears that patient expectations and preferences for a female obstetrician drove subsequent patient satisfaction. In the study, male obstetricians conducted longer visits and engaged in more dialogue than their female counterparts. They were more likely to check that they have understood the patient, using paraphrasing and interpretation, and to use orientations to direct the patient through the visit. In addition, male physicians expressed more concern and partnership than female physicians. Even though patient satisfaction was generally sensitive to physicians' communication, over and above the explanatory power of particular communication and patient variables, female physician gender predicted higher patient satisfaction ratings.

The relationship of physician gender to patients' ratings of the physicians' emotional responsiveness was especially strong and may reflect sensitivity to gender expectations as women are generally perceived as more emotionally communicative than males (J. A. Hall, 1984). This judgment was made despite the empirical evidence in the study that male physicians, in fact, engaged in more emotionally focused exchange. The consequences of this type of unfair judgment is reflected in the plight of male obstetricians. As noted earlier, not only do men face discrimination in choosing obstetrics and gynecology residency programs, but they continue to be discriminated against even after completing their training. In February of 2001, the *New York Times* published a story describing the plight of a male obstetrician fired from his practice ostensibly because of his inability to compete with his female colleagues in attracting patients (Lewin, 2001). The physician sued the practice for gender discrimination, raising questions regarding the right of the practice to accommodate female patients who request female doctors at the expense of equally qualified male doctors.

The closing quotation of the story is especially telling as the physician remarked: "I think it's similar to certain fields where women have to work harder to prove themselves. Men in this field have to be more sensitive." Patients, for their part, will be similarly challenged to fairly evaluate their physicians based on the physician's performance and not simply the physician's gender.

What might the results reported in this chapter mean for male physicians? We do not suggest that all, or even most, female physicians are patient-centered and male physicians are not; there is far more common ground than there are differences in the communication behaviors of male and female physicians. Moreover, both male and female physicians who are skillful communicators may achieve time efficiencies that allow the delivery of high-quality, patient-centered care in even restricted time frames (Roter & Hall, 1995). Physicians have the capacity to improve their communication skills in meaningful ways through self-awareness, self-monitoring, and training. The potentially powerful impact of patient reciprocation of both communication style and affect in the medical visit is especially important to recognize, as recognition could help create positive exchanges and defuse negatively spiraling interaction patterns.

The challenge for a more positive transformation in the everyday practice of medicine includes the generation of gender-neutral social norms regarding patient expectations and judgments of physician conduct, as well as the establishment of medical practice norms that value communication skills and interpersonal sensitivity. Simply having more women in medicine will help contribute to a societal norm that does not inherently define doctor in gender-linked terms, but this will not be sufficient in itself to transform medical practice. Physician training in interpersonal skills emphasizing those aspects of communication identified in the growing evidence base of medicine can contribute to the definition of quality standards for interpersonal communication for all physicians.

Part II

What Usually Happens in Medical Visits

7

The Anatomy of a Medical Visit

It has been estimated that a primary care physician will conduct between 160,000 and 200,000 patient visits during a 40-year professional career (Lipkin, Putnam, & Lazare, 1995). A typical patient will visit a doctor several hundred times over a lifetime; if the patient is female, this number will increase several fold, as she is likely to visit doctors accompanying her children, her spouse, and her parents. Although some of these visits will last only a few minutes and others will last an hour or more, most of the complicated business of healing is accomplished in relatively short, sporadic meetings. And this does not include the myriad medical encounters that are not in person. The use of new technologies has transformed the provision of specialty services and consultations to patients in underserved, rural, or inaccessible areas, and has promoted the delivery of care through telemedicine and other remote systems, including the use of pharmacy and medical robots. The Internet has also expanded the routine ways in which doctors and patients communicate. Though most patients take telephone access to their physician for granted, some observers of medical culture anticipate that e-mail access will shortly become similarly commonplace (Delbanco & Sands, 2004; Ferguson, 1998).

In this chapter, the anatomical features of the medical visit will be presented: its structure, duration, function, content, and, to some extent, format. To this end, we will document how a doctor typically proceeds throughout a visit, how long a visit takes, what a doctor attempts to accomplish, what a doctor is likely to say, what a patient is likely to say back, and how patient access to physicians through e-mail may affect the nature of medical exchange. The descriptions presented in this chapter are based on actual observations of thousands of routine medical encounters. We have collected some of this material ourselves, and for the rest have relied on the work of a host of other researchers.

Direct observation of medical visits has not had a very long tradition. Despite intense interest, dating back to the days of Hippocrates, in the therapeutic encounter, it has only been since the late 1960s, with advances in recording technology, that the medical encounter has been systematically observed. Perhaps because of the physical exposure of the exam, there is an element of privacy to the medical visit that has discouraged the researcher's intrusion. But physical exposure is only one aspect of the visit that is considered private; discovery of illness, and the fears and vulnerabilities that may accompany it, are also intensely private. Legal structures and professional ethics have surrounded the visit to ensure that these discussions can be open and free from fear. Confidentiality is jealously guarded. In an emotional, physical, and legal sense, communications between doctors and patients and the documentation of these in patients' charts are treated as "privileged communications."

In light of the high regard and protective structures surrounding the privacy of the medical visit, it is surprising that physicians and patients are willing to have their visits studied at all. However, they usually are. Several large studies of routine medical interactions over the past 20 years or so (Byrne & Long, 1976; Levinson, Roter, Mullooly, Dull, & Frankel, 1997; Roter, Lipkin, & Korsgaard, 1991; Roter, Stewart, Putnam, Lipkin, Stiles, & Inui, 1997) report that fewer than 10% of the patients who were asked refused to participate. In smaller studies, we found a 10%–20% refusal rate—about what is expected in any research project.

What these patients and physicians are agreeing to, with assurances that their names or any other identifiers will not be used, is most often an audio or videotape recording of their entire medical visit. Occasionally, a nonparticipant observer, a researcher who observes or takes notes during the medical visit but who does not participate in any way, is present. Virtually all studies provide participants with the option to withdraw from the study, turn the recorder off for any period of time, or ask the observer to leave; however, this is rarely done.

Recordings are used to provide researchers with more than just a verbatim record of what is said during the medical visit; they also reveal the nonverbal communication that is so crucial to conveying and establishing the psychological tone of the encounter. Even when only voice recording is done, nonverbal qualities can be captured because coders are able to rate the emotional tone of each speaker during the visit based on an overall impression created by both what is said and how it is said; that is, the specific content of the dialogue and also the voice quality of the participants can be studied. Of course, when videotapes are made, an even richer record is available.

One may question whether the presence of an observer or recorder inhibits or changes what goes on between the patient and doctor. An infringement of the privacy of the medical visit, an invasion of its privileged communication, could somehow violate its very nature. This does not appear likely. Both patients and doctors report forgetting about the recording soon after the visit begins, and few have indicated that being recorded changed their visits in any way. Moreover, the diversity of both patient and physician behavior that was observed through these tapes reflects the frank and open manner in which they were made. Byrne and Long (1976) noted in their study that the many incidents of physician failure with patients make the likelihood of censored behavior unlikely. We have similarly concluded that the broad range of physician behavior evident in our meta-analyses (quantitative summaries) of the communication literature suggests that there is little conscious manipulation of behavior in any systematic way (J. A. Hall, Roter, & Katz, 1988; Roter, Hall, & Aoki, 2002).

Nevertheless, it still may be true that recorded visits capture "best behavior." The issue of performance bias in response to tape recording has been addressed in several studies (Coleman & Manku-Scott, 1998; Inui, Carter, Kukull, Haigh, 1982; Pringle & Stewart-Evans, 1990; Redman, Dickinson, Cockburn, Hennrikus, & Sanson-Fisher, 1989). All of these studies have found the effect to be minimal. Included among these studies is one comparing video recordings of physicians who were and were not informed that they were being recorded. There were no statistically significant differences in length of visit or in the number or nature of the problems discussed (Pringle & Stewart-Evans, 1990).

VISIT DURATION

Many readers will be surprised to learn that medical visits are longer than they were 10 years ago. Despite the widespread perception that patients have less time with doctors, Mechanic and colleagues have found that the average medical visit has increased between one and two minutes in duration over the past decade, and that this increase is evident in both managed care and fee-for-service practices (Mechanic, McAlpine, & Rosenthal, 2001). This does not mean that visits feel less hurried. Mechanic suggests that, on the contrary, visits may feel *more* time-pressured than in the past, despite the additional time, because physicians are expected to provide more preventive and counseling services than ever before.

The amount of time that patients spend with their doctors during a medical visit will vary depending on a whole range of factors other than the medical problem being addressed. As noted in our earlier chapter on physician gender, female physicians conduct longer visits (by about 10%) than male physicians, and female patients tend to have slightly longer visits than male patients. The visit duration also varies according to the doctor's specialty; visits to a family physician are likely to be shorter, by several minutes, than visits to an internist, and visits within managed care systems tend to be a couple of minutes shorter than those with physicians receiving fee-for-service payment (Mechanic et al., 2001). Other factors affecting visit length may be more surprising. A British study of appointment scheduling found that the time of day for which a visit is scheduled affects the amount of time the doctor spends with the patient (Byrne & Long, 1976). Patients seen early in the day had visits that were 10%–40% longer than the average visit, but patients seen during the late afternoon had visits that were 25%–50% shorter than the average visit. It was clear that early in the day the doctors were more relaxed and took more time with their patients, but by mid-afternoon the pressure to complete their patient schedule led to shorter visits. The doctors in the study were quite surprised at the findings; they were completely unaware of these differences.

It is interesting to note that U.S. medical visits are quite long relative to most European medical visits. Estimates of the average visit length for general practitioners in Europe range from 7 to 16 minutes; comparable U.S. visits average 17 minutes (Mechanic et al., 2001; van den Brink-Muinen, Verhaak, & Bensing, 1999). These numbers suggest that visit length may be a consequence of the characteristics of the national health system as much as national habits and medical care expectations.

Does the length of visit hold significance for the nature of the medical discourse? The answer is yes. Short visits are associated with less problem identification (Howie, Heaney, & Maxwell, 1997), fewer preventive actions undertaken (Howie et al., 1997; A. D. Wilson, McDonald, Hayes, & Cooney, 1992; A. D. Wilson, 1985), and less lifestyle or psychosocial discussion (Robinson & Roter, 1999). Many patients report greater ease in discussing problems and participating in decision making when the visits are longer (F. M. Hull & Hull, 1984; Kaplan, Greenfield, Gandek, Rogers, & Ware, 1996). However, it should be noted that the overwhelming majority of patients are satisfied with the time they get for their visits (Howie et al., 1997; Kaplan et al., 1996; Morrell, Evans, & Morris, 1986), and many studies have reported inconsistent or weak associations between length of visit and quality of care delivered (Carr-Hill, Jenkins-Clarke, Dixon, & Pringle, 1998; L. Ridsdale, Carruthers, Morris, & J. Ridsdale, 1989).

THE STRUCTURE OF THE MEDICAL VISIT

The medical visit unfolds in a predictable five-phase sequence: the opening, the history, the physical examination, patient education and counseling, and the closing. These visit segments are presented in interviewing textbooks as a rough organizational plan that acts to facilitate orderly and systematic progression through the many visit tasks (Cohen-Cole, 1991; Lazare, Putnam, & Lipkin, 1995). Despite its importance, there has been little systematic investigation of visit structure, and few studies have comprehensively addressed the duration or sequence of visit phases.

For this reason, we think it especially interesting to review relevant data, not previously published, regarding the visit sequence from the large 11-site study of primary care communication (collected by the Collaborative Study Group of the Task Force on the Medical Interview; see, for instance, Roter et al., 1991). We found that 77% of the more than 500 primary care visits studied included distinct and sequenced history, exam, and patient education and counseling phases. Of the remaining visits, 13% included some combination of history and exam phases without an educational/counseling segment; and the last 10% of the visits contained history and/or educational/counseling phases without a physical exam. The study assessed the proportion of all visit dialogue devoted to these phases as follows: 48% to the opening and history segment (combined); 16% to the physical exam; and 36% to education/counseling and the closing (combined).

Furthermore, an interesting pattern in terms of relative patient and physician contributions to the dialogue emerged across visit phases. Patients were most verbally active during the history segment of the visit, contributing almost half (48%) of the dialogue. This changed dramatically for the remainder of the visit; patients were least talkative during the physical exam, contributing 36% of the exam statements, and they were only slightly more active during the education/counseling segment, contributing 39% of the statements. The total amount of visit dialogue was not related to the amount of dialogue in any particular segment; however, more dialogue in one segment was related to less dialogue in another. For instance, history talk was substantially negatively correlated with patient education and counseling dialogue, and longer physical examination discussions were negatively related to discussion in both the history and education/counseling segments.

In the first of our studies of physician gender effects on the medical dialogue, we found not only that female physicians conduct visits with substantially more dialogue overall, but also that much of this difference appears during the history segment of the visit (Roter et al., 1991). Female physicians talked 40% more than male physicians, and patients of female physicians talked 58% more than patients of male physicians, during the history portion of the visit. No other significant differences in male and female physician dialogue were found for the other visit segments, although patients of female physicians contributed somewhat more dialogue to the exam segment than patients of male physicians. A great deal more detail regarding physician gender effects on communication is presented in Chapter 6.

The Opening of the Visit

Among the few studies addressing a specific phase of the visit are the well-cited study by Beckman and Frankel on the opening of the visit and the larger follow-up study performed some 15 years later (Beckman & Frankel, 1984; Marvel, Epstein, Flowers, & Beckman, 1999). In this work, the primary task of the visit opening was defined as the physician's solicitation of the chief complaint, marked by broad questions such as "What seems to be the problem?" or "What brings you to the office?" The opening is concluded when the physician elicits the details of a presenting problem; this also marks the transition to the history segment of the visit. The investigators found that only a minority of physicians, about one-quarter, resisted following up on a problem until a statement of all the patient's concerns was complete. The average length of time to transition from the opening to the history segment of the visit was less than 23 seconds (18 seconds in the first study). In those instances in which a patient was encouraged to continue after the first concern until all problems were noted, the average duration was 32 seconds (28 seconds in the first study). In no instances did a patient take more than two minutes to describe all of his or her concerns.

Both the original and the follow-up study came to similar conclusions: physicians are quick to redirect patients from presenting concerns (during the opening of the visit) to the history segment; this has the effect of limiting the full disclosure of all the patient's concerns. The investigators also found that, in about 20% of visits, patients spontaneously initiated a new concern after the completion of the history portion of the visit; new concerns were less likely to arise late in the visit if the physician had specifically asked whether the patient had more concerns during the opening.

The Closing of the Visit

In a somewhat parallel fashion to the elicitation of patient concerns in the opening phase of the medical visit, Barsky (1981) examined concerns surfacing as "hidden agendas" during the closing minutes of the visit. Barsky found that, although patients present medical concerns early in the visit, they wait for the "right" moment to present emotionally charged concerns and fears. When the opportunity for this disclosure is not presented early in the visit, sensitive concerns are more likely to be blurted out at the last possible moment, sometimes initiating a new discussion of symptoms or treatment during the visit closing.

Pursuing a similar line of inquiry, J. White and colleagues further investigated the closing moments of the visit (J. White, Levinson, & Roter, 1994). In this study, closure was defined as a brief focused segment, with defined tasks, generally following the patient education and counseling phase of the visit. Marker phrases such as "Okay, let's see you back in four or five months" and "If it's not getting better in a week, let me know" were used to demarcate the closing. The length of the closure phase of the visit averaged 1.6 minutes, or 10% of the length of the entire visit. This estimate, however, includes both usual visit closings and those that were prolonged for one reason or another. Three-quarters of the visits closed in less than one minute, but the remaining visits continued for as long as nine minutes.

Patients raised new concerns in 21% of the closings; for example, they brought up new symptoms or asked for a blood pressure check. In at least some of these cases, the physician elicited additional history by asking questions about symptoms or therapeutic regimen and re-examined the patient. Interestingly, fewer problems were raised during the visit closing when, earlier in the visit, patients and physicians more fully discussed the therapeutic regimen, when physicians oriented the patients to the flow of the visit (for instance, "Now I'm going to examine you and then we will have some time to talk about what's going on"), and when the physician asked about patient beliefs ("What do you think may have caused this problem?"). Visits in which coders globally rated physicians as being more responsive to patients had fewer late problems raised. This might be related to Barsky's suggestion that physician failure to facilitate patient disclosure is related to delayed problem presentation.

The Physical Exam Phase of the Visit

The length of the physical exam was timed in two primary care studies, one in the United States and the other in the Netherlands (Bensing, Roter, & Hulsman, 2003). To increase comparability, both studies focused on routine care of hypertensive patients. Not only were the U.S. visits substantially longer than their Dutch counterparts (16 versus 9 minutes), but the physical exam portion of the visit was longer as well (3.9 versus 2.2 minutes). The average proportion of the visit time spent on the physical exam, however, was similar in the two samples—about a quarter of the visit length. These numbers reflect a relatively small number of visits (23%) that had physical exams averaging almost 50% of the visit time. Interestingly, the proportion of exceptionally long physical exam visits was very similar in both the Dutch and U.S. samples.

Overall visit length was not related to the duration of the physical exam, which suggests that especially long physical exams are accommodated within visits by curtailing other visit phases, most probably the patient education and counseling segment, as suggested by the unpublished data from an earlier study, discussed previously.

THE FUNCTIONS AND CONTENT OF THE VISIT

Medical dialogue is the vehicle for the development of the doctor-patient relationship and the primary mechanism through which the work of the medical visit is accomplished. Using a functional heuristic, Table 7.1 expands upon earlier reflections on the three-function model of medical interviewing (Cohen-Cole, 1991; Lazare et al., 1995) to suggest four functions of the medical interview and their predominant interaction elements. These include data gathering, patient education and counseling, responding to patient emotions, and facilitating patient participation in the dialogue. The relative importance of the interviewing functions varies depending on the care setting, health status of the patient, nature and extent of the prior relationship, as well as other exigencies. Nevertheless, each interviewing function contributes in some manner in all visits. Although not discussed as an explicit interviewing function, the accomplishment of basic technical-medical tasks, such as physical examination, blood draws, and the administration of injections, are, of course, important to the delivery of quality care.

The complexity of the dialogue used to accomplish the visit's medical functions is daunting. Our reviews of this literature found some 250 unique communication variables derived from observations of patient-physician interactions (J. A. Hall & Roter, 2002; J. A. Hall, Roter, & Katz, 1987; Roter & Hall, 2004; Roter, Hall, & Katz, 1987; Roter et al., 2002). Virtually all of these variables, however, fit within the four functions of the medical interview mentioned earlier and reflected in Tables 7.1 and 7.2. (This basic framework was also used in our meta-analyses of physician-patient communication in relation to the physician's gender; see Chapter 6.)

PHYSICIAN TALK

The actual frequencies of each category listed in Tables 7.1 and 7.2 are displayed in Tables 7.3 and 7.4; the information listed in these tables combines to provide a quantitative portrait of the medical encounter. First, reviewing physician talk (Table 7.3), we found that physicians spend the most time on patient education and counseling. This includes all forms of information giving, as reflected by the subcategories listed in Table 7.1. For some physicians, this involves merely reciting of facts ("Your blood pressure is high today, 180/95"); counseling ("It is very important that you take all the medication I am prescribing—you have to get your blood pressure under control, and this medication will do it, but only if you take it as directed"); or directions and instructions ("Put your clothes back on and sit down—now, take these pills twice a day for a week and drink plenty of water"). Each of these has a different intent—to inform, to persuade, or to control (respectively). From our own work, it appears that the giving of facts comprises about half of this category, and both counseling and directing patient behavior contribute in equal parts to the remainder. The next chapter will be devoted to a deeper exploration of information and its importance in the medical visit.

Data gathering by physicians also accounts for a good proportion of the visit; this is usually done during history taking and mostly consists of closed-ended questions. Closed-ended questions are those questions for which a one-word answer, usually yes or no, is expected ("Are your leg symptoms worse after standing for several minutes?"). In contrast, questions that allow patients some discretion in the direction they may take in answering are open-ended questions ("Tell me about your leg pain—what seems to be the problem?"). Considering the complexities of diagnostic reasoning, patients are hard-pressed to know what it is about their symptoms or medical history that the physician might consider relevant to their current problem. The physician's questions provide the cues that patients use in deciding what it is they should tell the doctor.

Closed-ended questions limit responses to a narrow field set by the physician; the patient knows that an appropriate response is one or two words and does not normally elaborate any further. In contrast, open-ended questions suggest to the patient that elaboration is appropriate and that the field of inquiry is wide enough to include patient thoughts about what might be relevant. These two types of questions have very different implications for control of the medical visit; closed-ended questions imply high physician control of the interaction, while open-ended questions are much less controlling. Closed-ended questions are often posed as a method of hypothesis testing; it is assumed that, if a physician is on the right track, and has a fair sense of what the patient's problem is, closed-ended questions are efficient prompts to the patient to give the physician the information needed. Open-ended questions, on the other hand, are often suggested under hypothesis uncertainty. If the physician does not have a clear idea of the underlying problem, open questions can help orient him or her and provide a starting point. In routine practice, closed-ended questions far outnumber open-ended questions, by a factor of two or three to one; closed-ended questions are thought to be less time-consuming and more efficient at getting the physician the information needed to make a diagnosis.

Our own work on how physicians collect information from patients sheds some light on this issue. Contrary to the widespread practice favoring closed-ended questions, we found that open-ended questions prompted substantially

Table 7.1
Specific Variables Included in Physician Categories

I. Patient Education and Counseling

Gives information, gives opinions, gives suggestions, gives instructions, provides education, gives explanations, provides orientation, explains, discusses problem resolution, provides descriptions, discusses disclosure, answers patient's questions, discloses information on the following: the patient's condition, the nature of the illness, the cause of the illness, the symptoms of the illness, the diagnosis, current health treatment, non-medical treatment, medical treatment, self-care, physical activity, diet, health promotion, lifestyle

II. Data Gathering

Asks for information, obtains instructions, takes medical history, asks about compliance (open-ended and closed-ended questions), asks questions, asks for patient's questions, seeks patient's ideas

III. Responding to Patient's Emotions

Emotional talk: Agrees, shows approval, laughs, shows solidarity, gives reassurance, offers support, facilitates, encourages, shows empathy, calms patient, communicates in a positive manner
Negative talk: Disagrees, confronts, shows antagonism, shows tension
Social chitchat: Greets, makes nonmedical statements (social conversation), exchanges personal remarks, makes social remarks, makes casual conversation, discusses social/family matters

IV. Partnership Building

Asks for patient's opinion, asks for understanding, asks for suggestions, requests patient's questions, seeks patient's ideas, makes interpretations, reflects patients' statements, facilitates responses from the patient, makes acknowledgements

Table 7.2
Specific Variables Included in Patient Categories

I. Information Giving

Presents symptoms, answers questions, responds to instructions, describes problem-related experiences, gives suggestions, shares opinions, provides information

II. Question Asking

Asks for orientation, asks for opinions, asks for instructions, asks for suggestions, asks general questions, asks questions about medications, asks about treatment, asks about lifestyle, asks about prevention, asks about self-care

III. Expressing and Responding to Emotions

Positive talk: Laughs, expresses friendliness, shows solidarity, releases tension, agrees, shows approval
Negative talk: Shows antagonism, disagrees, shows tension
Social conversation: Greets, makes social remarks, uses introductory phrases, makes non-medical social conversation, makes family/social conversation (not psychosocial exchanges)

Table 7.3
Profile of Physician Interactions

Variable	# Studies	Range	Mean	Median	Weighted Mean	S.D.
Patient Education/Counseling						
	12	4–60%	35.5%	38.5%	24.8%	16.90
Data Gathering						
	12	6–40%	22.6%	22.5%	20.1%	9.61
Partnership Building						
	7	3–25%	10.6%	10.0%	8.8%	6.52
Responding to the Patient's Emotions						
Emotional Talk	10	1–31%	15.0%	14.5%	11.9%	9.27
Social Chitchat	6	5–10%	6.0%	5.0%	5.4%	1.83
Negative Talk	3	0.5–2.5%	1.3%	1.0%	2.3%	0.94

Table 7.4
Profile of Patient Interactions

Variable	# Studies	Range	Mean	Median	Weighted Mean	S.D.
Information Giving						
	9	28–67%	46.9%	54.0%	43.5%	14.50
Question Asking						
	9	2.6–14.5%	7.0%	6.0%	6.1%	3.53
Social Conversation	5	4–42%	13.4%	7.0%	5.7%	14.40
Positive Talk	4	11–23%	18.7%	20.5%	20.11%	4.92
Negative Talk	3	5–13%	8.3%	7.0%	9.5%	3.40

more relevant disclosure of information than closed-ended questions (Roter & Hall, 1987). Because standardized cases were presented by actors in the study, it was possible to calculate the effect of appropriate open-ended and closed-ended question use on the extent to which the standardized patient revealed relevant information about his or her compliance behavior. Both question forms elicited relevant information; however, open-ended questions did so far more effectively than closed-ended questions. Indeed, the correlation between open-ended questions and relevant disclosure was almost twice the magnitude of the correlation for closed-ended questions.

Responding to patient emotions comprises a smaller share of physician's talk (only half as much time as questions) and serves a variety of functions. Shared laughter, approvals, empathy, support, and reassurance all increase a positive bond between speakers. Social, non-medical conversation comprises a small portion of the interaction, and includes greetings, casual remarks, and niceties ("Hello, Mr. Waller, nice to see you—that was some baseball game last night"). This talk is important as a social amenity; it is usually positive, and people are accustomed to greetings and a certain amount of chitchat in most encounters, at least initially, to put people at ease and express some degree of warmth and friendliness.

Finally, negative talk, as is obvious from Table 7.3, is quite rare from physicians. This includes disagreements, confrontations, and antagonisms ("You've gained weight since your last visit, and I am disappointed in you—you're not really trying at all"). It is probably a good guess that, even though negative talk is not often made explicit by physicians, the intent is expressed and negative emotional messages are conveyed. Professional etiquette and training discourage unpleasantness and the high emotions that may arise from direct criticisms and contradictions. Our findings imply that physicians find other ways to express displeasure. Reprimands may be expressed as forceful counseling or imperatives on the need to follow recommendations better. For the unsuccessful dieter, for instance, this could mean exhortation for the patient to do better on his diet and follow a prescribed regimen. The physician may also express displeasure in an angry, anxious, or dominant tone of voice or by cutting patients off in various ways.

Partnership building represents the physician's attempts to engage the patient more fully in the medical dialogue. Asking specifically for the patient's opinion, paraphrasing what the patient has said to check that it was understood, or asking the patient if he or she understands what the physician said are explicit ways in which the patient may be drawn more fully into the medical dialogue. Another kind of physician statement, more aptly described as noises than words—uh-huh, aha, and ah—signals that the physician is attentive and eager for the patient to continue. In the study of visit openings that was mentioned earlier, it was found that the more a physician used these noises, the more likely he or she was to uncover fully the patient's major concerns and reason for the visit (Beckman & Frankel, 1984). As Beckman and Frankel noted, patients readily defer to the physician and are easily diverted from giving their thoughts. Attentive noises, however, encourage elaboration so that a patient's full agenda for the visit can be revealed.

PATIENT TALK

Patient talk is studied less often and less intensively than physician talk. For instance, in our descriptive summary of the communication literature, we found that physician interactions were investigated in twice the number of studies as patient interactions and that the number of communication variables noted in the physician studies was substantially greater than in the patient studies (Roter, Hall, & Katz, 1988).

Research clearly shows that patients almost always talk less than physicians do during medical visits. This is something of a revelation to physicians—they generally overestimate the amount of patient talk and underestimate their own talk. The relative amount of patient contribution to the medical dialogue averages around 40% (ranging, in our review, from 23% to 49%) (Roter et al., 1988).

As might be anticipated, more than half of patient talk is providing information, largely in response to physicians' questions, as reflected in Table 7.4. What is surprising, however, is how little interaction, some 6%, is taken up by patients asking questions. This is particularly troubling because many studies have demonstrated that patients often have questions they would like to ask but do not. It has been suggested that this reticence may reflect a reluctance to appear foolish or inappropriate or it may be that physicians, in myriad ways, signal that the time is not right to ask questions. Whatever the reason, it is relatively rare for patients to ask questions.

In the studies we reviewed, negative talk was seven times more common for patients than for physicians. It is notable how much more frequently patients directly contradict or criticize the physician than the other way around. Patients may be more direct in this regard than their physicians because they have fewer communication options; they cannot easily express their disagreements through lecture, counseling, or imperatives. Physicians may also cultivate a habit of not showing emotions, whereas patients may feel that the role of the patient permits and even requires them to freely express their feelings.

It is also noteworthy that patients also engaged in more positive talk than physicians. The expression of these emotionally laden statements generally marks greater interpersonal engagement. The patient is likely to have a far greater emotional investment in the proceedings than the physician, and this is expressed in both positive and negative terms.

NONVERBAL COMMUNICATION

Emotion—fear, shame, disgust, anger, confidence, affection—are as much a part of the communication involved in medical encounters as any of the categories of talk described earlier. However, just as a picture is worth a thousand words, emotion is most powerfully conveyed nonverbally. It is within this context that nonverbal behavior has a significant role in medical care. We define nonverbal behavior to include a variety of communicative behaviors that do not carry linguistic content (Knapp & Hall, 2005). Briefly, these include (among others) facial expressions; eye contact; head nodding; hand gestures; postural positions (open or closed body posture and forward to backward body lean); paralinguistic speech characteristics such as speech rate, loudness, pitch, pauses, and speech dysfluencies; and dialogic behaviors such as interruptions.

Both physicians and patients show emotions, sometimes in spite of efforts at suppression or masking. For example, both physicians and patients reveal their liking of each other, at least enough so that they can each pick up on it at greater than chance levels (J. A. Hall, Horgan, Stein, & Roter, 2002). Some of the emotional cues that are conveyed by patients reflect the presence of their illnesses. These include cues relating to physical pain (Patrick, Craig, & Prkachin, 1986; Prkachin, 1992) and to physical and psychological distress (J. A. Hall, Roter, Milburn, & Daltroy, 1996). Coronary disease is associated with distinctive vocal and facial expressions (J. A. Hall, Friedman, & Harris, 1986). Among patients with coronary illness, episodes of ischemia correspond with facial movements associated with anger (Rosenberg et al., 2001). Some of the cues expressed by a patient are inadvertently conveyed, while others are part of the patient's deliberate effort to convey the experience of symptoms and suffering to the physician—experiences that are difficult to express in words (Heath, 2002).

The evidence that emotions are shown in the medical visit implies that both physicians and patients judge each other's emotions. Each group does this to gain insight into how the other feels. For instance, in one study, physicians were asked to rate whether their patients liked them, and patients were asked to rate whether their physicians liked them; liking was defined as having feelings of warmth and friendliness, and an enthusiasm for seeing someone (J. A. Hall et al., 2002). Some degree of accuracy in judging their liking of each other was evident, and, while it was significantly greater than chance, it was still quite modest. It is interesting to note that the patients and physicians in these studies demonstrated about equal accuracy in predicting how much each was liked by the other, and the liking tended to be mutual (i.e., positively correlated between physician and patient). Although individuals may make explicit references to the quality of their relationship in words, this is rare. We believe it is much more common for feelings of liking, warmth, and enthusiasm to be conveyed, and reciprocated, through nonverbal behavior, such as voice tones, facial expressions, or body postures.

Physicians also use patients' affective cues in the diagnostic process, as well as in evaluating clinical progress and overall well-being. For example, physicians may elicit emotions to help make a diagnosis, such as in the case of expressive aphasia, or may look for certain nonverbal cues when concerned about a patient's possible depression or when estimating how much pain the patient is experiencing. There is research suggesting that primary care physicians generally do poorly at recognizing patients' emotional distress, perhaps because they fail to fully attend to emotional cues. The work of Bensing and colleagues supports this contention; physicians who gazed frequently at the patient were more successful in recognizing psychological distress, as measured by a standard screening instrument (Bensing, Kerssens, & van der Pasch, 1995). The implication of the study is that greater eye contact results in more effective reading of emotional cues, leading to better recognition of psychosocial distress. It is also possible that eye contact enhances listening skills and thus the ability to more accurately synthesize and interpret verbal and nonverbal cues of distress.

Although there are many ways in which physicians and patients may reciprocate behavior, analyses of voice quality and other nonverbal behaviors reveal an especially subtle, and possibly unconscious, demonstration of emotional reciprocity. Using electronically filtered excerpts of speech, J. A. Hall, Roter, and Rand (1981) found strong evidence that the voice qualities of doctors and patients were related to one another. Independent judges' ratings of emotions in separate tapes of doctors' and patients' speech showed that, when the doctor sounded angry, anxious, or contented, so did the patient (and vice versa). Thus, they mirrored each other's vocal affect. Similarly, Street and Buller (1987, 1988) found positive correlations between physicians and patients on verbal interruptions, illustrative gestures, body orientations, and gazing patterns.

Such correlations suggest several interesting questions. Does one participant set the tone and the other follow, or do they each reflect back the other's affect in a spiraling fashion? If the latter is true, we can imagine both positive and negative spirals. Of course the negative spiral is the most dangerous, and all the more so because individuals rarely appreciate that their own behavior has produced the other's response. Thus, the grumpy patient whose doctor responds grumpily will likely attribute the doctor's behavior to negative personal qualities or attitudes, without realizing that the doctor was simply responding in kind to the patient's own behavior.

MEDICAL EXCHANGES THROUGH E-MAIL

Not all medical exchange is face-to-face. Just as most patients take telephone access to their physician for granted, many observers of medical culture believe that e-mail will shortly become similarly commonplace (T. Delbanco & Sands, 2004; Ferguson, 1998). An online survey of 2,000 adults conducted by Harris Interactive (March 27 through April 2, 2002) reported that 90% of respondents who regularly use the Internet wanted access to their physicians online. Far fewer patients, however, are actually able to access their physicians online. A large national phone survey (more than 60,000 U.S. households) in early 2002 revealed that 6% of the respondents with Internet access used it to contact a physician or other health care professional (L. Baker, Wagner, Singer, & Bundorf, 2003). The proportion of physicians who have ever used e-mail to communicate with a patient is estimated at 25%; however, only 10% use it regularly (Manhattan Research, 2004).

Only a few studies have described the content of actual e-mail exchanges between patients and their physicians, and these studies suggest that e-mail is largely used to accomplish administrative tasks such as scheduling appointments, refilling prescriptions, and exchanging information (T. Delbanco & Sands, 2004; C. B. White, Moyer, Stern, & Katz, 2004). Because its use tends to be task-focused, some fear that e-mail may diminish the social, emotional, and psychosocial dimensions of care by reducing medical communication to brief, electronic exchanges; this raises the question of whether e-mail exchanges can be patient-centered (Baur, 2000).

Our own exploratory study of e-mail use provides some insight, and reassurance, in this regard (Roter, Larson, Sands, Ford, & Houston, 2006). A sample of 74 e-mail messages, accumulated between eight patients and their physicians, were coded. Three-quarters of the physicians', and slightly more than half of patients', statements were devoted to information exchange; the remaining communication was characterized as expressing and responding to emotions and acting to build a therapeutic partnership. We concluded that e-mail accomplishes informational tasks, but it is also a vehicle for emotional support and partnership. Furthermore, there may be some advantages to e-mail exchanges over in-person visits.

E-mail was the only form of interactive exchange dominated by patients, with patients making longer and more detailed statements than their physicians. There is some reason to suggest that simply being at home may free patients from the social constraints of the role of being patients and enable them to convey sensitive, embarrassing, or especially distressing information that may be withheld in face-to-face visits (Lazare, 1987). For instance, Strasser and colleagues describe a case study in which e-mail was used as a therapeutic tool by which a dying patient daily communicated her fears and concerns to the care team (Strasser, Fisch, Bodurka, Sivesind, & Bruera, 2002). The patient understood that there would be no response to these messages, but that they would be read and provide a way in which the care team could listen to their patient's concerns. E-mail "fit the patient's desire to control communication and possibly to interact on grounds other than the hospital territory, thus escaping from her and her physicians' roles" (p. 3353). In this instance, e-mail meaningfully enhanced the patient-centered nature of the care given to this patient.

STYLES OF MEDICAL INTERVIEWING

Communication style is an integrative combination of communication elements that reflects something more than a sum of its individual parts. Style in communication, as in dress or art or cooking, reflects an underlying consistency with which a repertoire of behaviors is expressed. We have found it useful in our work, as have other researchers exploring this issue, to characterize interviewing style as "doctor-centered" or "patient-centered."

A doctor-centered style tends to be task-focused and designed to facilitate the efficient accomplishment of the visit's biomedical and administrative functions: the gathering of sufficient information to test clinical hypotheses in order to make a diagnosis and recommend treatment, and the need to have the visit proceed quickly and efficiently. In contrast, a patient-centered style has become the shorthand reference for an appreciation of the patient's illness experience (as opposed to disease and pathology), the patient's perspective and preferences in care, and the very nature of the therapeutic relationship and humanity of patients and physicians (Mead & Bower, 2000). Examples of physician communication behaviors that are patient-centered include information giving and counseling in both the biomedical and psychosocial domain, open-ended questions, paraphrasing and interpreting patient input to ensure understanding of the patient, asking for the patient's opinions and expectations, checking that the patient understands the information that is conveyed, and making socioemotional statements of concern, reassurance, empathy, and approval. We believe that this is true whether the doctor-patient exchange occurs during a medical visit, on the telephone, or through e-mail.

8

Giving and Withholding Information: The Special Case of Informative Talk in the Medical Visit

Part of medicine's mystique is that it is written and often communicated in code. To make matters worse, the code has two forms: the scientific, anatomical, and technologically correct usage of terms to describe body parts, body processes, medical procedures, and medical treatments, and a second, even more impenetrable shorthand for these things used by doctors in hospitals. Ironically, there is some evidence that physicians themselves have trouble understanding this code (Christy, 1979). The use of "medicalese" and the various forms of medical jargon and code persists despite its problematic nature. Indeed, it is not unusual for a patient to feel alarmed and confused after leaving the doctor's office because of failures to understand what the doctor was talking about.

It is a good guess that a doctor will use at least one unfamiliar medical term in any given visit. In their pioneering work in this area, Barbara Korsch and her colleagues (Korsch, Gozzi, & Francis, 1968) found that the pediatrician's use of difficult technical language and medical shorthand was a barrier to communication in more than half of the 800 pediatric visits that were studied. Mothers were often confused and unsure of terms used by the doctor to describe what was wrong with their children and what the doctor was going to do about it. Although one mother asked the doctor to "repeat what he said in English," this kind of confrontation appeared infrequent; for the most part, mothers did not ask for clarification of unfamiliar terms. Fear of appearing ignorant was the reason most often given for not asking what technical terms meant. The investigators suggested that some patients may think it flattering to have the physician think that they understanding difficult and unfamiliar language, and this makes it even harder to admit otherwise (Korsch et al., 1968).

Others have similarly reported both patient confusion and reluctance to ask for clarification. Going so far as to suggest a "communication conspiracy" to be common in medical visits, Svarstad (1974) noted that physicians in her study generally spoke as though their patients understood them and the patients acted as though they understood their physicians—even though this was far from the truth. In only 15% of the visits in which an unfamiliar term was used did patients actually tell doctors that they did not recognize or understand the term. Most often, the patients simply remained silent.

Our research confirms that technical terms are still commonly used in medical encounters. In one study of 100 primary care visits, an average of 5 different technical terms, usually a reference to a body part, procedure, symptom, or biochemical marker (e.g., temporomandibular joint, sigmoidoscopy, dysrhythmic, tricyclics) were found in a typical visit. Although a substantial degree of variation was observed in different physician styles, most often technical terms were used without explanation and when lay terms could have been easily substituted. Less experienced physicians (including medical residents) were more likely to use medical jargon than were the more senior physicians, but the junior physicians were also more likely to give patients an explanation of the term. Thus, less experienced physicians may both "show off" their knowledge of big terms *and* feel the need to tell the patient what they mean. An alternative interpretation of the seniority effect may be that younger physicians feel more on a par with patients and feel less of a need to talk down (by simplifying their language) than higher ranking (or older) physicians do.

The use of technical jargon is even more pronounced in genetic counseling sessions. Transcript analysis of 150 genetic counselors in simulated client sessions (including both cancer and prenatal cases) found that an average of 11 different genetics-related technical words (e.g., syndrome, mutation, susceptibility) were used in a typical session, and they were repeated an average of 10 times. Counselors differed significantly from one another; some counselors used only one or two technical terms during each session, while others used as many as 21. Nevertheless, on the whole, familiar words could have been easily substituted for many of the terms, but only a minority of counselors did so (Roter, Erby, et al., 2006). The impact of medical jargon on patient comprehension and recall of information conveyed during the simulated sessions was examined in this study in an indirect way. Subjects who were similar to the simulated clients in the sessions (women with a family history of cancer or a mother over the age of 35) were recruited to watch a videotape of a genetic counseling session and complete a variety of post-session questionnaires. Among these was a measure of information recall and comprehension. The researchers found that the more the counselor used technical terms, the less information subjects were able to recall after watching a video-tape of the counseling session. These findings suggest that the use of technical terms and jargon may be distracting or confusing.

The use of medical terms in relation to medical diagnosis is one area in which patients may derive benefit from having their physicians use medical terms. Ogden and colleagues designed an interesting study in which primary care patients were asked to evaluate two hypothetical medical problems labeled either in lay terms (such as stomach upset and sore throat) or in medical terms (such as gastroenteritis and tonsillitis) (Ogden et al., 2003). The investigators found that patients rated medically labeled problems as more deserving of sympathy and as a more legitimate excuse for loss of work days than problems that had been labeled in lay terms. Respondents also indicated greater confidence in the physician when the medically labeled diagnosis was presented. Furthermore, a diagnosis labeled in lay terms was associated with a negative evaluation of the patient; respondents more often thought that the patient should not have brought the problem to the doctor and that the problem was related to something the patient had done him- or herself. The authors cautioned that the current shift toward lay language may inadvertently lead to diminished confidence in physicians and a greater assignment of patient self-blame.

Doctors are not completely unaware of the problems that patients have with technical terms and explanations. Several studies indicate that, if anything, physicians generally *underestimate* what patients understand (McKinlay, 1975). In a particularly telling study, physicians were asked to identify terms they thought their patients would have difficulty understanding. The list was found to be far more restrictive than a parallel list of problematic words generated by patients. This did not mean that the physicians were careful to restrict their communication. In fact, an analysis of the words actually used by these physicians when with patients found that they used many of these terms they did not expect their patients to understand. In the case of genetic counselors, we found a somewhat similar phenomenon. The greater the number of technical words that were used, the less effective the counselor felt he or she was in educating the study client (Roter, Erby, et al., 2006).

Why would doctors use terms they thought their patients would not understand or why might genetic counselors educate clients in a way that they felt was not optimally effective? Several reasons come to mind. The first takes the view that physicians may believe that most patients are unprepared to evaluate and comprehend the complex information they may receive (Freidson, 1970). After all, most patients have not gone to medical school and lack the years of training necessary to approximate the sophistication of a physician. Even if medical terms could be put into lay language, translation is a time consuming and difficult task. Furthermore, it has been argued that patients are too upset at being ill to be able to use the information they get in a manner that is meaningful, even if put in lay terms. This perspective is especially argued in respect to information related to a new diagnosis or a life-threatening condition.

A more cynical and self-serving perspective can also be taken; information is power and an informed patient is a possible threat to the physician's professional status and control of the therapeutic situation. Inasmuch as an informed patient may question a medical decision or outcome, maintaining a patient as uninformed affords protection from the likelihood of uncovering mismanagement or mistakes (Barber, 1980; Skipper, Tagliacozzo, & Mauksch, 1964). As further discussed in Chapter 9, assertive or aggressive patients who press for informational details are perceived by physicians to be a litigation risk, and sometimes refused care on this basis (Studdert et al., 2005).

Malpractice suits based on inadequate informed consent have damaged, but certainly not made obsolete, the longstanding medical tradition that favors discretion by a physician in disclosure of information to patients over the duty to tell the truth. Supported by various codes of medical ethics and by the legal doctrine of therapeutic privilege, physicians may choose to withhold relevant information from patients in cases where they believe that the information may do the patient some harm. By virtue of their expert training and knowledge, some physicians maintain they can best determine what is best for their patients, or so the argument goes; the decision to disclose certain kinds of information to a patient is as a much a professional decision as is the making of a diagnosis (Holder, 1970).

The problem is that physicians and patients often disagree as to the likely outcome of disclosure, and consequently what is in the patient's best interest. A study of the information preferences of patients and information-giving practices of neurologists underscores this point (R. Faden, Becker, Lewis, Freeman, & A. Faden, 1981). In general, patients preferred detailed and extensive disclosure of almost all risks even when they were quite rare. Further, information about alternative therapies was highly valued by about 90% of the respondents. By contrast, the physicians indicated that they were likely to disclose only risks with a relatively high probability of occurrence; only about half of the doctors thought patients would want information about alternative therapies. Moreover, the physicians were much more likely to agree with the view that detailed disclosure of information regarding drugs would decrease positive placebo effects, increase side effects through the power of suggestion, and decrease compliance. Patients expressed a completely different view. They believed more information would increase their confidence in the drug, improve their compliance, and generally serve to make them feel more comfortable with the therapy they were receiving.

Especially telling was how physicians responded to the question "If you felt that telling a patient something about the drug would make the patient very upset and anxious, what would you do?" Sixty percent of the physicians surveyed indicated that they would inform the patient anyway; 20% indicated that they would inform another member of the family; and 20% said that they would withhold the information completely. Most patients (80%) indicated that they would want to be given the information, and those who had some reservations about it indicated that they would want another member of their families to be informed. None of them indicated that they would want the information withheld altogether (Faden et al., 1981). Clearly there is a communication gap.

Doctors appear particularly reluctant to give bad news. A recent survey of oncologists suggests that this practice is widespread (Lamont & Christakis, 2001). When doctors were asked what they would tell cancer patients in an outpatient hospice if they insisted on knowing their survival prognoses, 23% said they would not supply an estimate; 37% said they would communicate a frank prognosis; and 40% said they would communicate an inaccurate prognosis. Of the latter, two-thirds said they would convey an optimistically biased prognosis. It is at this juncture that the fine line between maintaining hope and preserving trust is broached; many physicians feel that they have inadequate communication skills to do either (Ford, Fallowfield, & Lewis, 1996). Despite years of research suggesting that dying patients very often suspect the truth even when their prognoses are withheld, and that nondisclosure is even more psychologically devastating than disclosure (Kubler-Ross, 1969), the practice of nondisclosure, while declining, is still commonplace. In some instances, physicians are responding to a request by the patient's family to withhold disclosure, sometimes so that family members themselves can deliver the prognosis, or because family members believe that the prognosis would be devastating for psychological or cultural reasons (Carrese & Rhodes, 2000). While this subject is primarily studied with respect to cancer, there are enough other examples in the literature to consider that the tendency to diminish the extent of a negative prognosis is evident across specialties (Quine & Pahl, 1986; Quint, 1972). While the primary motivation for less-than-frank disclosure of bad news may be the maintenance of patient hope, there are other motivations that are more self-serving for the physician. Protection from the sadness that bad news is likely to create for the doctors themselves is often noted, as well as the more pragmatic management benefits associated with avoiding emotional scenes and the need to comfort patients, tasks that are viewed as onerous and time consuming (Quine & Pahl, 1986; Quint, 1972).

One consequence of physician control of information is patient passivity; the less information provided, the less the patient is likely to engage in the dialogue by asking questions or initiating concerns. While patients appear to wait for the physician to take the initiative in providing explanations before asking questions, physicians sometimes take the patient's reserve as an indication of lack of interest or incompetence and tend to shortcut pertinent disclosure or discussion (Cartwright, 1964; Pratt, Seligmann, & Reader, 1957). One conclusion that may be drawn from this is that physicians have primary control over patient participation in the medical visit by providing at least a minimal framework of information within which the patient can arrange thoughts and formulate questions. Though there is merit to this argument, not all patient questions are derived from medical or technical knowledge. It is easy to imagine that personal experience, anxiety, fright, and the observation of others provide a basis for patient questioning. Patients are not dependent on physician-provided explanations of illness to formulate the kinds of questions described above. Yet, patients do not ask many questions of any kind.

The first studies in this area found that patients seldom made forceful demands for information from their physicians, although a substantial proportion of patients would frankly admit to an interviewer that they would like more information about some fundamental aspects of their condition (Kutner, 1972; Reader, Pratt, & Mudd, 1957; Tuckett, Boulton, Olson, & Williams, 1985). For example, Tuckett et al. (1985) found that 75% of patients interviewed in their study indicated that they had specific doubts or questions during their medical visits that they did not mention to the doctor. For the majority of the patients, questions were withheld because they were fearful of the doctor's reaction. Patients expressed dread of having the doctor think badly of them or misunderstanding their motivation for questioning. They were quite anxious that the doctor might think they were second-guessing the doctor's judgment. Further, few patients thought that their doctors actually wanted them to question them, and patients felt an urgency about the time they were taking from the doctor's really needy patients. Moreover, feeling hurried clearly interfered with the patient's ability to gather his or her thoughts and clearly articulate questions. For these patients, the lack of question asking was far more likely to reflect a lack of skill in clearly articulating ideas or questions than lack of interest.

Lack of patient skill in question asking has been observed in other studies, as well. In fact, one researcher observed that the main communication problem physicians faced was their patients' inability to clearly express themselves (Hughs, 1982). In response to an open-ended opportunity to speak, the investigators found that patients just ran out of words and the doctor took the floor to prevent an uneasy silence.

When patients ask questions, their doctors virtually always provide them with answers (Boreham & Gibson, 1978; Roter, 1977; Svarstad, 1974). Further, patients who are more verbally active during the visit by offering their own explanations or thoughts about their condition, asking questions, or expressing doubts are treated differently from those patients who are not as active (Tuckett et al., 1985). Active patients were more likely to receive the kind of practical information that was helpful in making decisions.

PATIENTS' RECORDS AND BEDSIDE CASE PRESENTATIONS

Although physicians may be disinclined to communicate all relevant details regarding a patient's condition or prognosis, they are likely to be conscientious about noting the particulars in the patient's medical chart. However, patients have not traditionally had easy access to their own medical records. An editorial in the *New England Journal of Medicine* in 1973 made the somewhat radical recommendation that legislation be passed to require that a complete and unexpurgated copy of all medical records, both inpatient and outpatient, be given to patients routinely and automatically (Shenkin & Warner, 1973). Even more controversial was the suggestion that not only should patients view their records, they should be invited to be a coauthor (Fischback, Bayog, Needle, & Delbanco, 1980). What seemed revolutionary several decades ago is now commonplace. The longstanding debate regarding chart access has been effectively ended with the passage of the Health Insurance Portability and Accountability Act of 1996 (HIPAA). HIPAA mandates that patients be able to see and get copies of their records, and that they may request amendments if there are errors.

While some investigators have warned that patient access to medical records could cause undue anxiety, confusion, or even embarrassment, most studies in the area demonstrate minimal harm and modest benefit (S. E. Ross & Lin, 2003). Among the benefits, the chart has been found to help fill the gaps in communication between doctor and patient, act as an educational tool for patients, reduce suspicion that the physician is keeping something from patients, and enable patients to act more autonomously in making judgments and choices about their care (S. E. Ross &

Lin, 2003). Although patients tend to be interested in reading their records when it is offered, and the medical record can surely provide information in a straightforward and uncensored way, few patients make a formal request for their records. The convenience and portability of electronic patient records may transform this situation. As more programs are instituted in which patients are encouraged not only to maintain a current copy of their medical record but also to use it as an educational and motivational tool to enhance self-care and health promotion activities, the notion of a coauthored medical record may be closer to reality. As discussed in more detail in Chapter 10, interventions using the medical record can help patients and doctors talk more productively to one another, advance a true patient-physician partnership, and contribute to a variety of health benefits.

Another indirect route by which patients may become privy to their own medical information is through medical rounds. Despite concern that patients are discomforted and made anxious and confused by bedside rounds, and a general trend away for its use, Lehman and colleagues found that there were few negative reactions and that some patients benefited from the process (Lehmann, Brancati, Chen, Roter, & Dobs, 1997). The patients who had been randomly assigned to have bedside rounds reported that their doctors spent significantly more time with them—twice as much—while they were in the hospital than the doctors spent with other patients. This suggests one of two things: that patients actually see very little of their physicians in the hospital, so that rounds substantially increase contact time, or that rounds increase the impression that the physicians are spending more time with their patients. In any case, patients with rounds tended to report that their physicians provided a more adequate explanation of the patients' problems, and these patients appeared to have a more positive hospital experience than the other patients.

Half the patients experiencing bedside presentations reported that it had helped them understand their illnesses. However, it should also be noted that many patients reported that too much confusing medical terminology had been used during the rounds. Ratings in this regard differed by both patient race and level of education. In general, African American patients had more favorable perceptions of the presentations than Caucasian patients did (after statistically adjusting for age, gender, and education), and African American patients were more likely to think that their physicians had provided adequate explanations of their problems. In a similar manner, better educated patients were far less likely to complain about confusing terminology being used during rounds and were far more likely to say that their doctor had adequately explained tests and medications than less well educated patients.

In a *New England Journal of Medicine* editorial accompanying the Lehman study, Thibault (1997) argued that there are compelling reasons to attempt to reverse the decline in rounds. Bedside rounds provide a window into the processes of care, and not just the technical processes but also the interest and concern that doctors, and others that are part of the care team, have for the patient. One indicator of that concern is time and information—both of which are conveyed during rounds. This does not imply that bedside rounds cannot be improved. They certainly can. Vocabulary can be simplified and patients can be included in the presentation in a more meaningful and substantive way. Moreover, there are pedagogical reasons to continue the tradition of bedside rounds. As articulated by the renowned diagnostician William Osler, there should be "no teaching without a patient for a text, and the best teaching is that taught by the patient himself" (Osler, 1903, quoted in Lehmann et al., 1997, p. 1150).

THE INTERNET AS A HEALTH INFORMATION SOURCE

In many respects, and especially in regard to the provision of medical information, the Internet, as many commentators have noted, has changed everything. This applies in spades to health information. According to the Pew Internet and American Life Project (S. Fox & Fallows, 2003), fully half of the American adult population has used the Internet at least once to search for health information. Among people who are regular Internet users, 80% say that they use online sources to seek health or medical information. This is not an everyday activity but something that is undertaken when health issues or questions arise.

Health information obtained online is used in a variety of ways, including: to research a diagnosis or prescription, prepare for surgery or to find out how best to recover from surgery, to get tips from other caregivers and patients about dealing with a particular symptom, and to obtain emotional support from others sharing a common health or medical problem. The great majority of those who look for health information online say that what they find is useful, at least most of the time, and that what they learn is new to them (S. Fox & Fallows, 2003). Even more impressive is that the information obtained online is reported to have improved the way the survey respondents take care of themselves, especially in terms of what they eat and how they exercise. Almost 70% indicated that their last online health search affected their decision about how they might treat an illness, whether to visit a doctor, ask new questions, or get a second opinion. Indeed, one in three of online health seekers who find relevant health information bring it to their doctor for a "quality check" (S. Fox, 2003).

As more and more patients come to their medical visits well informed, or at least well supplied with advice and information pertinent to their medical problems, physicians are confronted with the task of trying to establish which pieces of information are valid and which are not. This can be, of course, a time consuming endeavor. How time consuming this activity is may vary depending on the physician's specialty and the kinds of information patients are likely to bring. Within the context of oncology visits, a survey of practicing oncologists estimated that physicians spend 10 additional minutes discussing the online health information that patients bring with them (Helft, Hlubocky, & Daugherty, 2003). The oncologists expressed mixed feelings in regard to this information, reporting that it can simultaneously affect patients in both positive (more hopeful and knowledgeable) and negative (confused and anxious) ways. It also has a mixed effect on physicians. Forty-four percent of the oncologists in the survey reported that they have had difficulty, even if only occasionally, discussing Internet information with patients, and 9% reported that they have occasionally felt uncomfortable when patients brought Internet information to them for discussion (Helft et al., 2003). Patients reported mixed physician receptivity to their presentations of online information; some physicians were reported to welcome it, while others expressed irritation and defensiveness (S. Fox & Fallows, 2003).

As a result of Internet access, as well as the information dissemination efforts of many patient advocacy groups, patients are sometimes better informed than their physicians. This is particularly evident when the patient's medical condition is rare. As noted by one respondent to the Pew survey, "as the parent of a child with a very rare neurological syndrome, the Internet was vital to putting the pieces of a puzzle together. It saved my son months of struggle when I found a diagnosis prior to the neurologist he was seeing, who openly admitted she had only heard of the syndrome but never treated a child with [Landau-Kleffner syndrome]" (S. Fox & Fallows, 2003, p. 7).

More than half of Internet health searches are conducted on behalf of someone else. In this regard, it is not surprising that women, the better educated, the affluent, and adults under the age of 65 are more likely to conduct health topic searches online than others. As discussed in Chapter 4, this is the same demographic profile of patients most likely to ask their doctors questions during medical visits. For others, especially users with low or marginal literacy skills, Internet access and use of online health information can be especially problematic (Baur, 2004). Commonly used single-word search strategies, such as searches for "health" or "cancer," that are employed by Internet users with low literacy skills can result in an overwhelming number of listings, making it difficult to distinguish credible information sources from commercially placed advertisements. Moreover, since the information on most Web sites is presented at a high reading level, interpretation of information is especially problematic (Baur, 2004).

DRUG INFORMATION

In the 1980s, a national, random survey of 1,104 persons, conducted within 2 weeks of receiving a new prescription, revealed that information given to them about their drugs was sparse. Particularly revealing were the findings that (1) 35% of the patients said they didn't receive any information at all from either their doctors or pharmacists about the drugs prescribed for them; and (2) 75% of the patients did not recall being told by their physicians what possible side effects the prescribed drugs might have (R. W. Miller, 1983). Despite these obvious gaps in information about their drugs, patients were not at all active in seeking this information out. Only 2 to 4% of the patients said they asked any questions about their prescriptions while in their physicians' offices. This changed dramatically following the 1997 FDA publication of guidelines to industry on direct to consumer (DTC) advertisements (Aikin, Swasy, & Braman, 2004). Although critics fear the DTC advertisements lead to unnecessary, expensive, and potentially harmful overprescribing of drugs, it has also been argued that the campaigns serve a useful educational function for both patients and physicians in encouraging discussion of symptoms and conditions that may be poorly recognized or highly stigmatized (Kravitz, 2000).

Two FDA surveys of patient attitudes and behaviors related on DTC advertising over the past few years (1999 and 2002) found mostly positive effects, although the trend seems to indicate a decline in consumer enthusiasm over time (Aikin et al., 2004). The survey targeted adults who had had a recent medical visit, and it asked a host of questions regarding the impact of DTC advertising on patient care. While only 4% of the respondents said that they visited their doctors because of a DTC advertisement, 33% took advantage of the visits to ask their doctors about an advertised drug. Half of the visits in which patients asked whether a prescription was available to treat a condition resulted in a prescription. While 10% of the patients were reluctant to talk to their doctors about a DTC-advertised drug for fear of implying distrust, 43% felt the ads helped them have better discussions with their doctors. On the whole, patients seemed to have benefited from the DTC advertisements; 32% felt that the ads helped them make better health decisions, and 18% said that the ads helped remind them to take their medications. Some patients (17%) were less positive about the ads and said that the ads caused them some anxiety about their health.

The FDA also conducted a parallel survey of physicians in 2002 (Aikin et al., 2004). The vast majority (85%) of surveyed physicians reported that drug-related discussions were frequent. When asked to remember a specific, recent visit in which a patient had asked about an advertised drug, three-quarters of the physicians indicated that their patients asked thoughtful questions because of the DTC exposure. However, 41% indicated that their patients were confused about the advertised drug's effectiveness. Primary care physicians were more frequently asked about DTC drugs than specialists, and they also reported feeling "somewhat" or "very" pressured to prescribe a drug. One-quarter of the physicians thought that DTC advertising led to tension in the doctor-patient relationship. All in all, the physicians were evenly divided in their overall impressions of DTC marketing; about equal numbers of physicians indicated that it had a positive effect, a negative effect, or no effect at all.

NOT ALL PATIENTS WANT INFORMATION

Social psychologists have argued that some individuals may benefit more than others from being highly informed or involved in their own treatments, while, for other patients, detailed information may actually increase anxiety through information "overload" (Mills & Krantz, 1979). For instance, S. M. Miller and Mangan (1983) found that it was useful to classify patients as information avoiders or information seekers to predict a patient's psychophysiological response to varying levels of information while undergoing a painful medical procedure. The researchers found that a patient's level of anxiety was lower when the level of information given to the patient was consistent with the patient's coping style; information avoiders did better with less information, and information seekers did better with more information. These findings provide a context for interpreting the responses of 15% of the patients interviewed in the British study by Tuckett and colleagues (1985), mentioned earlier, that indicated that the patients had not asked questions of their doctors because the patients were not interested—they felt that knowing about medical matters was "not for them."

Additional insight into the distinction between avoiders and seekers is provided by Steptoe, Sutcliffe, Allen, and Coombes (1991), who found that, although all patients who reported that they understood little about their conditions desired additional information, information avoiders generally reported higher understanding of their conditions and greater satisfaction with doctor-patient communication than information seekers. However, scores on objective knowledge tests were lower for the avoiders than for the seekers. The authors concluded that information avoiders reported a better understanding of their conditions not because of superior factual knowledge but "because their coping style led them to avoid further direct information that might highlight their predicament" (Steptoe et al., 1991, p. 628). Despite better understanding, information seekers were nonetheless less satisfied with communication and felt there was more to know about their conditions that they would like their doctors to share with them.

THE TWO-WAY FLOW OF INFORMATION

As is evident in this chapter, most researchers have conceptualized the informative event as a unidirectional flow of information from physician to patient—either stimulated by patient question asking or as information spontaneously given by the provider to the patient. However, there is a broader perspective on informative events in the medical visit that challenges the assumption of unidirectional flow. Effective information exchange is an interactive, two-way process, and, within these exchanges, the usefulness of the information a patient gets is very often contingent on the information the patient provides.

A patient spends most of his or her time during a medical visit providing information to his or her physician, largely in response to the physician's questions (mostly closed-ended questions) about the patient's medical condition. But this kind of information is incomplete. Giving a patient the opportunity to "tell his or her story" in an open manner, with minimal direction by the physician, can act to further the understanding, of both provider and patient, of the patient's condition and his or her experience. The reflection and insight that can arise from the telling of the story can move the exchange to a deeper and more meaningful level.

A second important information realm that patients only infrequently share with their physicians (and about which physicians infrequently inquire) is their "explanatory framework." This refers to the patients' interpretations of how and why they are sick, what will make them better, and what they hope the doctor can do for them. This kind of insight can provide the physician with a starting point for meaningful exchange. Knowing where patients are, in terms of their beliefs and theories, is essential if the provider hopes to attach any true relevance to the information given to the patient. Otherwise, information giving in the medical dialogue can be reduced to "two parallel monologues" in which patient and physician are both talking at cross-purposes and in two different languages (Mishler, 1984).

Moreover, information exchange conveys more than just substantive meaning. Research suggests that patients attribute positive affective motivation to a physician who is informative; the physician who takes time to inform patients fully is seen as sincere, concerned, interested, and dedicated

(Roter, Hall, & Katz, 1987). There is also evidence that physicians attribute positive characteristics to patients who are more verbally active in their visit, viewing them as more interested, concerned about their health, and intelligent.

Where do we go from here? One suggestion arising from the preceding discussion is that it is not sufficient simply to encourage physicians to be more informative or to train patients to ask more questions. That view takes doctor-patient interaction out of its context and strips away much of its dynamic productivity. Rather, it is important to appreciate the tremendous power of permitting a patient to orient his or her physician to the patient's "lifeworld"—to tell the patient's stories and share the patient's experiences, understanding, theories, and concerns about health (Mishler, 1984). It is this process that is informative for both the patient and the physician and from which important questions will freely arise and comprehensible information be derived.

Part III

Prospects for Improved Talk

9

Consequences of Talk: The Relationship between Talk and Outcomes

Researchers interested in the consequences of medical communication have largely focused on patient satisfaction with care and adherence to doctors' recommendations. Dissatisfied patients are less likely to return for visits, more likely to switch doctors and health plans, and more likely to initiate malpractice litigation than satisfied patients. Dissatisfaction, because it implies low trust, also undermines the nonspecific healing mechanisms implied in placebo and suggestion effects. And a dissatisfied patient almost by definition will miss out on the rapport and reassurance that is part of a good doctor-patient relationship.

Satisfaction is also linked to patient behavior because more satisfied patients are more likely to follow medical recommendations. Medical recommendations run the gamut from taking a single pill or following a complex drug regimen, to seeking preventive care and returning for follow-up appointments, or modifying aspects of lifestyle. Noncompliance with recommendations jeopardizes the patient's health and well-being, interferes with the doctor's therapeutic efforts, and leads to wasted health resources (DiMatteo & DiNicola, 1982).

Although not as commonly studied as satisfaction and adherence, there is a small and extremely important body of work that has linked doctor-patient communication to other measures of outcome, including indicators of patient health status (Kaplan, Greenfield, & Ware, 1989; Stewart, 1995).

Included among these measures are physiologic indicators such as levels of glycosylated hemoglobin (HbA1c) in the blood of diabetic patients and blood pressure in hypertensive patients. In addition, such measures as functional status (the patient's sense of his or her ability to perform usual daily routines) and a patient's overall sense of well-being and emotional coping have been linked to elements of the medical dialogue.

Finally, there are a few studies that have explored how physicians are affected by factors associated with the way in which they relate to patients and perform their work. Among these outcomes are physician satisfaction and the likelihood of becoming involved in medical malpractice litigation. An appreciation for these outcomes is underscored by the relatively high levels of physician stress and burnout, particularly in specialties associated with rising malpractice rates, and the medical workforce shortages made worse by increasing numbers of physicians taking early retirement.

It should not come as a surprise that many of the predictors of patient satisfaction also affect physician satisfaction. As we have stressed earlier in this volume, the communication of emotion is highly reciprocal. The positive regard associated with patient satisfaction with care and judgments of good performance, interpersonal rapport, and personal warmth and affection, are all likely to inspire physician satisfaction and similar feelings of liking. The opposite is true as well; critical judgments and perceptions of rejection or disregard also inspire similarly negative emotions. As will be discussed in this chapter, not only are patient and physician satisfaction and liking related to one another, but when these measures of a positive interpersonal and professional relationship are absent, patient compliance is lowered, therapeutic effect is diminished, and physician risk for malpractice litigation is heightened.

PATIENT SATISFACTION

Although studied often, the patients' perspectives on care have not always been highly regarded by the medical profession or researchers. Patients' judgments have been disparaged because of patients' supposed ignorance of the technical aspects of medicine and its jargon, their tendencies to be taken in by charlatans with good bedside manners, and their purportedly distorted views of what is important in medical care. Distortion is, of course, in the eye of the beholder. As patienthood takes on more consumerist qualities, and the medical system becomes more competitive, health care will cater more to what its managers believe patients want. The question, however, is what do patients want?

Perhaps the most common misgiving of the medical profession in regard to patients' evaluations of care is that they are thought to be unable to distinguish good from poor technical care—that is, the skills of diagnosis and treatment. We cannot say definitely how true or untrue this assumption is.

Nevertheless, some studies do suggest that patients can be appropriately sensitive to variations in quality and are more satisfied when quality is high. An example is a study of patients who came to an emergency room for treatment of burns (B. S. Linn, 1982). Physicians' technical performance was measured by researchers who scored the medical record for whether appropriate actions were taken. When the physicians performed better in these strictly "medical" tasks, their patients were more satisfied than when they performed worse. Although this study suggests that patients recognize good care when they see it, no one yet knows the limits of patients' abilities to make such discriminations (and there certainly are limits, for no one could expect a lay person to understand many of the finer points of medical science).

Research has definitely shown that patients have reasonably accurate perceptions of the interpersonal manner of the physician and can report the extent and nature of communication received from the physician. Moreover, patient satisfaction studies have reflected patients' abilities to recognize variations in medical care. In these studies, patients are not always asked, literally, about their "satisfaction." Sometimes they are asked instead to describe their care, and the investigator infers from these descriptions how satisfied they are. For example, agreement with the statement "My doctor answered all my questions fully" would be assumed to indicate high satisfaction because it is assumed a patient would want this to happen.

We know that there are differences in the behavior of medical residents versus more experienced physicians. The younger doctors have been shown to behave more competently, both technically and interpersonally, to engage in more nonmedical talk, and to conduct longer visits (J. A. Hall, Roter, & Katz, 1988). Other research shows that patients like it when their doctors have these traits. It is therefore not surprising to learn that patients are more satisfied, on average, with medical residents (J. A. Hall & Dornan, 1988a).

Table 9.1 shows characteristic items that might be used to measure patients' satisfaction. These are arranged, from top to bottom, to reflect the relative frequency with which these different aspects of medical care are asked about in research. Most often, patients are asked about their satisfaction with the humaneness or interpersonal qualities of their doctors, and least often about their satisfaction with the attention given to personal (not medical) problems or problems of living (J. A. Hall & Dornan, 1988b).

Patients are generally rather satisfied with the doctor overall, and with the doctor's humaneness, technical competence, and the health outcome of care. These elements received the highest patient ratings (ranks 1 through 4, respectively) out of 11 satisfaction elements in an analysis of over 107 published studies (J. A. Hall & Dornan, 1988b). Intermediate rankings, 5 through 7, were given to facilities, continuity of care, and access to care, respectively. The lowest ranks, 8 through 11, were found in

Table 9.1
Patients' Satisfaction with Medical Care: Sample Items

Item	Aspect of Medical Care
How satisfied are you with . . .	
. . . the respect accorded you by your doctor?	Humaneness
. . . how carefully your doctor listened to what you had to say?	
. . . the explanations given you by the doctor?	Informativeness
. . . the answers you got to your questions?	
. . . the doctor's performance overall?	Quality
. . . the quality of care you received today?	
. . . the health maintenance organization you belong to?	Overall
. . . your stay in the hospital?	
. . . the expertise of your doctor?	Technical Competence
. . . how thoroughly your doctor examined you?	
. . . how long you waited in the waiting room before seeing the doctor?	Organization
. . . the way the receptionist treated you?	
. . . how long it takes you to get an appointment?	Access
. . . how far from your home your doctor's office is?	
. . . your ability to pay for good medical care?	Cost
. . . the amount charged by your doctor for a visit?	
. . . the appearance of the clinic?	Facilities
. . . how modern the equipment is?	
. . . the pain relief you experienced?	Outcome
. . . the resolution of your medical problem?	
. . . your ability to see the same doctor each time you need one?	Continuity
. . . the continuity of care you receive at this clinic?	
. . . how much attention the doctor paid to problems at home or at work?	Psychosocial Care
. . . how much the doctor let you tell about any anxiety or depression you've had lately?	

Note: These questions might be answered on a rating scale that goes from 1 to 6,
where 1 = very dissatisfied, 2 = moderately dissatisfied, 3 = slightly dissatisfied,
4 = slightly satisfied, 5 = moderately satisfied, and 6 = extremely satisfied.

regard to physicians' informativeness, medical care cost, bureaucracy (including how long patients wait at the doctor's office) and, finally, at the bottom, physicians' attention to psychosocial problems.

The relative satisfaction rankings may reflect actual performance of the medical system, wherein some aspects of care may be emphasized over others, for example, technical skills compared with psychological support. Seen in this light, greater relative satisfaction for technical quality could mean that the health care systems emphasize technical performance to the relative neglect of patient needs that fall outside of a biomedical definition of health. These would include intellectual needs to be informed, psychological needs to be reassured and seen in the context of both social and biomedical problems, and economic needs for affordable health care and the avoidance of long waiting times (J. A. Hall & Dornan, 1988b).

The questions in Table 9.1 might be useful for readers to think about during, and after, visiting a doctor. They may also be useful for a doctor to think about as an aid in taking the patient's perspective in the visit. The exercise of thinking systematically about what the doctor does and does not do, and how one reacts to it, tells not only about the doctor but also about one's own expectations and values. This can be especially interesting for those who pay repeated visits to the same doctor or facility, for then ratings can be compared between visits.

Although in Table 9.1 all the questions refer to one's own doctor or recent experiences, sometimes the questions used in research refer to doctors or medical care in general. Most people score as more satisfied when describing their personal care than when describing care in general. Though this is not logically possible (everyone's care can't be above average), it is a common bias in how people evaluate ego-relevant aspects of their lives. For instance, people believe they are more happily married than average and are better drivers than average. Strong needs to maintain a positive self-image and a sense of personal control lead people to exaggerate the positive nature of things that are personally important. The need to look good or justify oneself is particularly strong when the issue in question involves choice, such as when one has chosen one's doctor or one's setting of health care.

Investigators often think of patient satisfaction as a multifactorial concept—meaning that there are distinct domains of satisfaction, such as those listed in Table 9.1. However, in practice, these domains tend to be highly correlated with each other, suggesting a "halo" effect whereby patients do not discriminate greatly between these domains. Thus, one's degree of satisfaction or dissatisfaction seems to spread across domains. When domains do emerge as distinct, the distinction that emerges tends to be between technical and interpersonal aspects of care (Hagedoorn et al., 2003; Marshall, Hays, Sherbourne, & Wells, 1993; Roter, Hall, & Katz, 1987).

Patient Correlates of Patient Satisfaction

In their meta-analysis (i.e., quantitative review) of studies that looked at patient sociodemographic characteristics as predictors of satisfaction, J. A. Hall and Dornan (1990) reported some results that are more surprising for what they are not than for what they are. Unlike earlier conclusions based on more limited reviews, the meta-analysis did not find any overall relationship between satisfaction and the patient's gender, ethnicity, or income. While several patient characteristics were related to satisfaction, these relationships were weak. Being older, having less education but a higher social status occupation, and being married were minor predictors of satisfaction.

Even though male and female patients do not systematically differ in their levels of satisfaction, the behavioral correlates of satisfaction are often different for male and female patients. In a study of 648 routine medical visits, male patients' satisfaction was significantly more positively correlated with social conversation, overall friendliness, and positive utterances than female patients' satisfaction was (J. A. Hall & Roter, 1995). In that study, there were not enough female physicians to break the analysis down further. J. A. Hall, Irish, Roter, Ehrlich, and Miller (1994b) included equal numbers of male and female physicians and patients in a study of general internal medicine. Two notable findings were that for the pairing of male patient with male physician, more psychosocial talk by the physician was strongly negatively correlated with satisfaction, whereas in the pairing of female patient with female physician, the exact reverse was the case, with the difference being highly statistically significant. Similarly, in pairings involving one or more males in the physician-patient dyad, more verbal interruptions were negatively correlated with satisfaction, whereas in the female-female pairing more interruptions were positively correlated with satisfaction. Both of these findings indicate that the same behavior can take on dramatically different meanings, and possibly different impact, depending on the gender of speaker and listener.

This is not to say that there are no important patient characteristics predictive of satisfaction. In this regard, patient health status is worthy of special note. Patients who are healthier are more satisfied than those who are less healthy, in both outpatient and inpatient settings, whether health be defined in terms of physical disorders or emotional distress (J. A. Hall, Feldstein, Fretwell, Rowe, & Epstein, 1990; J. A. Hall, Horgan, Stein, & Roter, 2002; Jackson, Chamberlin, & Kroenke, 2001; Krupat, Fancey, & Cleary, 2000). It appears that both the patient's intrinsic state of mind (which will be more negative when the patient is sicker) as well as how the patient is treated by the doctor can contribute to this effect (J. A. Hall, Milburn, Roter, & Daltroy, 1998). Certainly sicker patients (especially those with chronic conditions) interact more frequently with the medical care system and therefore have many more opportunities to experience bad medicine or upsetting behavior on the part of health care providers. Those who experience more negative events because of more frequent trips to the doctor could certainly have lower overall satisfaction than those who visit less often.

Just this point has been demonstrated by a large survey of patients and doctors conducted in the early 1980s. The researchers found that patients who had suffered from a chronic condition for many years were more knowledgeable about what constitutes good medical practice for that condition and were more critical of the care they received than were less experienced patients (Haug & Lavin, 1983). Being sick and/or dissatisfied may of course establish its own cycle, with such patients conveying more negativity to their physicians, which is then reciprocated. Our research indeed found that doctors had less liking for their patients who had worse physical and emotional health (J. A. Hall, Epstein, DeCiantis, & McNeil, 1993; J. A. Hall et al., 2002).

Communication Correlates of Patient Satisfaction

Audiotapes and other objective records of doctor-patient interaction, as well as patient reports, can be used to explore factors associated with higher and lower satisfaction. Studies of this kind reveal that the social climate established in the visit, through both verbal and nonverbal behavior, are major determinants of satisfaction according to many individual studies and reviews of the literature (J. A. Hall, Roter, & Katz, 1988; J. A. Hall, Harrigan, & Rosenthal, 1995; Ong, de Haes, Hoos, & Lammes, 1995; T. L. Thompson, 1994; S. Williams, Weinman, & Dale, 1998).

Satisfaction is increased when physicians spend more time with patients, show more nonverbal interest, lean forward more, engage in more nods and gestures, use more eye contact, establish a closer interpersonal distance, read the medical chart less, treat patients in a more partner-like manner, use more positively toned words (such as statements of agreement), use fewer negative words (such as criticisms), and engage in more social conversation (such as greetings and nonmedical chitchat). On the patient's side, higher levels of activation also are associated with improvements in satisfaction (Bertakis et al., 1998).

Nonverbal skill has also been studied by DiMatteo and her colleagues (DiMatteo, Taranta, Friedman, & Prince, 1980; DiMatteo, Hays, & Prince, 1986). In these studies, physicians' skills in nonverbal communication were measured using standardized tasks. One task measured how accurately they could recognize emotions in videotaped faces and voices; another measured how accurately they could express themselves emotionally through facial expression and voice tone. This research showed that the patients of doctors with more developed nonverbal communication skills were the most satisfied. At this point, one can speculate on what the high- and low-scoring doctors did that influenced their patients. We would guess that the more sensitive and expressive doctors interacted with patients in a way that was more attuned to the patients' needs. Perhaps they used their faces and voices more effectively to communicate empathy, or they were able to detect patients' feelings and thoughts that were not expressed through words. A patient who hesitates to speak about a problem, who is nervous or frightened, or who is angry, may convey these feelings nonverbally in ways that only a nonverbally sensitive physician can pick up. The physician is then in a better position to respond constructively.

Both communication style and nonverbal skill may contribute to perceptions of physician dominance, and a number of studies find that greater physician dominance predicts lower satisfaction, whether dominance is measured objectively (as in, a higher ratio of physician to patient talk; Bertakis, Roter, & Putnam, 1991) or in patients' ratings of physician dominance (M. K. Buller & D. B. Buller, 1985; Burgoon et al., 1987) (see review by Kiesler & Auerbach, 2003) or in assessments of vocal tone (J. A. Hall, Roter, & Katz, 1987; Roter, Hall, & Katz, 1987). Indeed, physician dominance is also related to the likelihood that a physician has been involved in a malpractice claim, as discussed later in this chapter.

The interpersonal climate is not the only factor that predicts satisfaction. One of the strongest predictors, in fact, among variables measured during the medical visit is how much information is given to the patient. Such information could be on diagnosis, the causes and course of a disease, or on possible treatments and what they entail. Patients who get more information are more satisfied than patients who get less (J. A. Hall et al., 1988; Jackson et al., 2001; Krupat, Fancey, & Cleary, 2000). This speaks to the high value placed on information by patients. The correlation of information to satisfaction could reflect not only a patient's desire for information per se; it could also indicate how patients feel about doctors who give more information. Patients may reason that a doctor who bothers to give more information is nicer or more concerned about them as people. Thus, two values may operate simultaneously—the value placed on medical information, and the value placed on having a humane and involved physician.

The way in which a doctor gathers information and the nature of the questions that are asked are also related to satisfaction. Whereas psychosocial questioning is very well received by patients, there is evidence that more questioning on biomedical topics is associated with lower satisfaction (Bertakis et al., 1991; Roter et al., 1987). At least two interpretations are possible. One is that more biomedical questioning by the physician occurs when the patient's health is worse, and, as discussed later, poor health is associated with lower satisfaction. Another interpretation is that more biomedical questioning by the physician is indicative of greater physician dominance, with the questions (which are most often of the closed, yes-no type of question) reflecting greater physician control over the dialogue; as noted, patients do not generally like physicians who are very dominant.

In addition to individual elements of interaction, physicians' overall styles of communication have been related to patient satisfaction. The patient-centered interviewing style, one in which the patient's point of view is actively sought and input is facilitated through open expression of concerns and question asking, is positively associated with patient satisfaction (Stewart, 1984; Roter et al., 1997). In a similar vein, M. K. Buller and D. B. Buller (1985) found that patients' reports of an affiliative style, composed of communication behaviors designed to establish and maintain a positive relationship between physician and patient, such as friendliness, interest, empathy, a nonjudgmental attitude, and a social orientation, predicted patient satisfaction to a much greater degree than a more dominant communication style.

These results also point to the kinds of physician behaviors patients do not want. Krupat, Rosenkranz, et al. (2000) found that patients were less satisfied when their physicians disagreed with attitude items such as "Patients should be treated as if they were partners with the doctor, equal in power and status." Those investigators also tested the important hypothesis that optimal outcomes occur when the physician and patient share congruent values about the balance of power. Satisfaction was particularly low when the patient placed higher value on shared power than the physician did.

Most research on patient satisfaction has been conducted in primary care outpatient settings. But there is a growing body of research in oncology that seems to indicate findings similar to those found in primary care. For example Ong, Visser, Lammes, and de Haes (2000) found that cancer patients' satisfaction was related to the affective quality of the consultation. Like most patients, those with cancer typically want more information than they get, are unsure of their diagnoses and prognoses, and are unsure of what diagnostic tests are needed and what they mean; indeed, oncologists themselves report being stressed by their poor training in communication, as described later in this chapter (Fallowfield & Jenkins, 1999).

A smaller amount of attention has been paid to studying communication issues for hospitalized patients, some of whom of course also have cancer. Consistent with what is known about outpatients, hospitalized patients are often unhappy with the amount of information they receive and they complain of inadequate time talking with nurses and doctors, not being told about hospital routine, not being told whom to ask for help, and not getting enough information about postdischarge care (Delbanco et al., 1995; Krupat, Fancey, & Cleary, 2000).

It should not come as a surprise that many of the predictors of patient satisfaction also affect physician satisfaction. As we have stressed earlier in this volume, the communication of emotion is highly reciprocal. The positive regard associated with patient satisfaction with care and judgments of good performance, interpersonal rapport, and personal warmth and affection, are all likely to inspire physician satisfaction and similar feelings of liking. The opposite is true as well; critical judgments and perceptions of rejection or disregard also inspire similarly negative emotions. As will be discussed in this chapter, not only are patient and physician satisfaction and liking related to one another, but when these measures of a positive interpersonal and professional relationship are absent, patient compliance is lowered, therapeutic effect is diminished, and physician risk for malpractice litigation is heightened.

Many of the physician behaviors that predict patient satisfaction suggest the way people act when they like someone. Indeed, research shows that, when doctors liked their patients more, their patients were more satisfied with them (J. A. Hall, Epstein, DeCiantis, & McNeil, 1993; J. A. Hall et al., 2002; Like & Zyzanski, 1987). Patients of doctors who liked them more were more satisfied even a year later and were less likely to have thought about changing doctors during the year (J. A. Hall et al., 2002).

PATIENT COMPLIANCE

The first major academic symposium on patient compliance was held at McMaster University in 1974. While individual researchers had documented poor patient compliance with treatment regimens prior to then, it was at this meeting that the magnitude of the problem became evident. Since then, hundreds of studies and literature reviews have been conducted in this area to identify predictors or correlates of patient compliance (DiMatteo, 2004). Patient compliance is now widely recognized as a critical link to effective treatment and successful management of a broad array of acute and chronic diseases. As a result of increased physician awareness of compliance as a clinically relevant concern, DiMatteo found (in the largest quantitative synthesis of this literature done to date) that the rate of patient compliance is generally improving. Studies conducted after 1980 yielded an average compliance rate of 75%, representing an improvement of 13 percentage points over the rates found for studies published before that period. This is a clinically relevant change reflecting an increasing awareness of the role of compliance in influencing medical outcomes.

Again and again, the most important contribution to patient compliance with drug prescriptions appears to be the patient's understanding of the illness, the rationale and importance of the drug therapy, and the instructions for use. However, full discussion of these points in the medical visit is, in fact, quite rare. Examining the physicians' verbal instructions to patients during medical visits in which drugs were prescribed, Svarstad (1974) found no discussion at all for almost 20% of the drugs and no information about the purpose and/or name of the drug in one-third of the cases. Advice on how long to take the drug was given in only 10% of the visits and how often to take the drug was mentioned in fewer than one out of five visits. These findings are not atypical; full and clear information about drugs is not very commonly given and there is not convincing evidence that the situation has changed very much in the thirty years since the Svarstad study. (A guide to a full discussion of drugs is provided in Table 9.2.)

Patients need to understand the treatment recommendations, believe in them, and have the ability to follow them. When they don't understand what they are to do or doubt a recommendation's usefulness, they ignore it; and when circumstances or supports are lacking, they are less likely to follow through as recommended (DiMatteo, 1994; DiMatteo & DiNicola, 1982; DiMatteo, Reiter, & Gambone, 1994). When the doctor offers more information, more positive talk, and less negative talk, and asks fewer questions overall (but more questions about compliance in particular), the more compliant a patient is likely to be (J. A. Hall et al., 1988). The association of less question asking to more compliance is consistent with research that found that question asking was inversely related to information giving (J. A. Hall et al., 1987). We believe that it is not only the substantive nature of the information given to patients that enhances patient compliance, but the attribution of caring and humaneness given to an informative physician by patients.

There is evidence that emotion transmitted through the doctor's tone of voice had an important effect on the patient's likelihood of following the doctor's recommendations. For instance, hostility in a physician's tone of voice in speaking about alcoholic patients predicted failure of the patient to go to an alcoholism treatment center (Milmoe, Rosenthal, Blane, Chafetz, & Wolf, 1967). Presumably, the patient noticed the doctor's hostility and rejection in the tone of voice during the medical visit, and responded by rejecting the doctor's suggestion for further treatment, even though that treatment was with other doctors in a different facility.

Our own research on physicians' voice tone similarly found a connection between the doctors' tone of voice and patients' subsequent behavior. We found that certain combinations of voice tone and actual words used by the doctor were related to patient satisfaction and appointment keeping (J. A. Hall, Roter, & Rand, 1981). Other research found that physicians' sensitivity to expressed emotion was significantly related to their patients' appointment-keeping patterns; the more sensitive physicians had fewer appointment cancellations that were not rescheduled (DiMatteo et al., 1986). We believe

Table 9.2
Medication Checklist

The following points or issues should be discussed when any drugs are prescribed.

1. Purpose and rationale for the medicine

2. Likely effect to be gained by taking the medicine and/or consequences of not taking the medicine

3. Name of the medicine

4. The amount of drug to be taken in a single dose

5. Total number of doses to be taken daily

6. Timing or sequence of doses

7. How the dose should be taken (with food, milk, etc.)

8. Maximum amount of the drug that can be used in one day (as with drugs to be taken as needed)

9. Length of time for which the medicine should be used

10. Other medications, specific foods, or activities that should be avoided

11. Proper storage techniques

12. Possible or likely side effects

Also, questions about drugs prescribed in previous visits are important in order to check that regimens are being followed correctly, if modifications are necessary, and if any side effects have occurred.

the notion of reciprocity is operating in these studies. Physicians affect patients by their expressions, and these, in turn, seem to influence patients' feelings of satisfaction, as well as patients' actual behaviors, such as keeping appointments.

A second area in which patient cooperation with physician recommendations is apparently lacking is in relation to lifestyle change. Adherence to physicians' recommendations in regard to smoking, weight control, diet modification, exercise, and alcohol restriction is far less complete than is adherence to drug regimens. These are, of course, difficult habits to change. Nonetheless, they are critical contributors to the chronic diseases, and responsibility to reduce these health-threatening habits is widely recognized as within the physician's purview.

Physicians, well aware of the smoking-disease link, believe that they have an obligation to counsel patients about harmful lifestyle habits (S. Goldstein, Fischer, Richards, A. Goldstein, & Shank, 1987). Yet, only two-thirds of physicians surveyed reported that they routinely advise their smoking patients to quit, and fewer than one-fourth offer any kind of systematic advice to their patients about quitting or refer them to outside sources of help for smoking cessation (Orleans, 1985). The situation regarding weight, exercise, and alcohol is even worse.

This lack of active involvement by physicians in an area they readily acknowledge as extremely serious is attributed to a variety of factors, most notably pessimism regarding effectiveness in motivating patients to change long-standing habits. Despite many physicians' own reservations regarding their effectiveness, physician recommendations are indeed taken quite seriously by patients. A number of studies have shown that the single most important reason people give for quitting smoking is concern over their health, and those who quit for health reasons or in response to physician advice are more likely to make repeated attempts and to remain off cigarettes (Orleans, 1985). The following statistics demonstrate that physicians are, in fact, more successful than they think they are: the national annual quit rate is 2–3%, whereas most studies in which physicians provide even minimal advice to patients show double and triple that rate. For the most part, this advice is given in a rather off-hand manner, taking a few minutes of time and without any consistent follow-up. When doctors make a special effort to counsel their patients to quit, particularly patients with some condition made worse by smoking, such as lung or heart disease, success in quitting is greater than 10 times the annual rate, from 30 to 50%.

An interesting study of how much talk during the medical visit is actually devoted to issues of prevention was undertaken by Freeman (1987). Freeman noted that, although the majority of physicians in her study said that they routinely talk about such health promotion issues as diet, exercise, drug and alcohol use, and family dynamics with their patients, this discussion was infrequent in the 200 visits she observed. When health promotion issues were broached during the visit, they were almost always extremely short references that were quickly passed over. Moreover, doctors seemed most comfortable with lifestyle talk when it was directly tied to a specific medical condition, as when the doctor related diet and weight control to diabetes management or smoking cessation to an episode of bronchitis.

Discussion was more awkward when health promotion talk was not tied to a specific condition, and in these instances, the discussion tended to occur toward the end of the visit. Doctors seemed somewhat embarrassed to be bringing up such topics as alcohol use or smoking and these comments sounded somehow "off the record" or not really a part of the business of the visit. Alternatively, the physician broached these subjects in a somewhat joking manner, perhaps anticipating patient rejection of prevention ideas. A Swedish study of lifestyle counseling in medical visits similarly found physicians uncomfortable with these tasks. Though Swedish doctors more often introduced the topics of smoking and alcohol than their American counterparts, the discussion was equally characterized as awkward, shallow, and fragmentary (Larsson, Saljo, & Aronsson, 1987).

Our own analysis of lifestyle talk, however, produced somewhat different results (Russell & Roter, 1993). We analyzed audiotapes of over 400 interactions between adult, chronic disease patients and their physicians in a variety of practice settings to explore the content, frequency, intensity, and dynamics of health promotion discussions during routine primary care medical visits. There was evidence of health promotion discussion in more than half of the audiotapes reviewed. Forty percent of the medical visits reflected some discussion about diet/weight control, at least twice the frequency of all other topics. Physical activity and stress were addressed with about equal frequency in 20% and 17% of the visits, respectively. Discussion of cigarette smoking was less frequent than the preceding topics, averaging about 11%; cigarettes were discussed almost twice as often as the least common topic, alcohol consumption (6%).

In those visits in which lifestyle topics were discussed, the exchange lasted an average of 4.5 minutes, or 20% of the total visit's time. Nearly 60% of the discussions went beyond the perfunctory to include attempts to counsel and/or encourage behavior change. To some extent, the difference between this report and others may be a function of changing times. As health promotion continues to gain prominence in both patient and physician consciousness, the changes in counseling frequency may reflect both greater patient demand for these services as well as greater physician comfort with promotion topics.

A patient's rejection of, or inconsistent adherence to, a doctor's recommendation is not a random occurrence. Surely all the responsibility for noncompliance cannot be laid to rest on the physician's shoulders; however, it is clear that in regard to drugs and lifestyle recommendations, in particular, messages are not conveyed in nearly as consistent and persuasive a manner as is desirable. If physicians do not make the effort to convey fully the importance of the recommendations they make, and provide some guidance for the behaviors they advocate, patients cannot be expected to fulfill them faithfully. Again, our notion of reciprocity is operable. Patients, we believe, will more fully comply with recommended behaviors when they believe that the doctor is serious about them. This message can be best conveyed to patients by physicians fully communicating their belief in the recommendations they make by taking the time to inform and counsel their patients about them.

Physiological Outcomes and Quality of Life

It is one thing to argue that good doctor-patient communication leads to higher patient satisfaction and even compliance with recommendations, but quite another to link communication to specific health outcomes. However, this link has been established in both hospital and outpatient studies. Doctor-patient communication has been associated with improved recovery from surgery, decreased use of pain medication, and shortened hospital stays (Mumford, Schlesinger, & Glass, 1982), as well as physiological changes in blood pressure and blood sugar (Bertakis et al., 1998; Kaplan et al., 1989; Schillinger et al., 2003).

In her comprehensive review of this literature, Stewart (1995) found strong evidence linking physician-patient communication to a variety of patient health outcomes, including emotional health, symptom resolution, functional status, physiologic measures (i.e., blood pressure and blood sugar level), and pain control. While the review was organized by fitting the effective communication elements in the studies to two phases of the visit (history taking and discussion of the management plan), the communication elements can also be related to key functions of the visit, including informativeness, partnership building, and emotional responsiveness, as described below (Roter, 2000b).

Being informative is a powerful communication function that is clearly linked to health outcomes. When the physician gives clear information, especially when coupled with emotional support, psychological distress is reduced (Roter et al., 1995), symptom resolution is enhanced (Haezen-Klemens & Lapinska, 1984), and blood pressure is reduced (Orth, Stiles, Scherwitz, Hennrikus, & Vallbona, 1987). When physician informativeness is coupled with the provision of informational packages and programs (particularly for patients undergoing radiation or surgery), pain is reduced (Egbert, Battit, Welch, & Bartlett, 1964), function is improved (Johnson, J. E., Nail, Lauver, King, & Keys, 1988), and mood and anxiety are improved (Rainey, 1985).

Visits that are participatory and contribute to the development and expression of active partnerships also have better health outcomes. Asking questions about patients' understanding of the problem, concerns and expectations, and perception of the impact of the problem on the patient's functioning was associated with symptom resolution (Haezen-Klemens & Lapinska, 1984) and reductions in patient anxiety (Evans, Kiellerup, Stanley, Burrows, & Sweet, 1987). When physicians encouraged patients to ask questions, patient anxiety was reduced in gynecology patients (S. C. Thompson, Nanni, & Schwankovsky, 1990) as were role and physical limitations in chronic disease patients (Greenfield, Kaplan, & Ware, 1985; Kaplan, Greenfield, & Ware, 1989; Greenfield, Kaplan, Ware, Yano, & Frank, 1988).

In visits in which the patient perceives a full and open discussion of the problem has taken place, symptom resolution is facilitated (Headache Study Group of the University of Western Ontario, 1986), and when the doctor and patient agree about the nature of the problem and the need for follow-up, both problem and symptom resolution is enhanced (M. J. Bass et al., 1986; Starfield et al., 1981). Finally, physician willingness to share decision making by giving patients the opportunity to choose among treatment options is associated with reductions in anxiety and depression, especially among cancer patients (Fallowfield, Hall, Maguire, & Baum, 1990).

Visits that are responsive to the patients' emotional state are also associated with positive health outcomes in both the physical and emotional domain. Physician probing explicitly about feelings and emotions and physician expression of support and empathy were associated with a reduction in psychological distress (Roter et al., 1995) and symptom resolution (Haezen-Klemens & Lapinska, 1984).

Finally, visits that are facilitative in helping patients effectively communicate their stories, express the full spectrum of their concerns, and ask questions, are associated with positive health outcomes. Specifically, when patient expression of feelings, opinions, and information was facilitated, there were improvements in physical and social role limitations (Greenfield et al., 1985), health status, functional status, and blood pressure control (Greenfield, Kaplan, Ware, Yano, & Frank, 1988; Kaplan et al., 1989). When the patient took the initiative for obtaining information (and fulfilling his or her informational agenda), physiological status (improvements in blood pressure for hypertensive patients and hemoglobin A1c for diabetic patients) and functional status were enhanced (Greenfield et al., 1985; Greenfield et al., 1988; Kaplan et al., 1989).

Stewart concludes her review by suggesting that improvements in communication require a shift in the balance of power between physician and patient. However, she notes that this shift should not be a full pendulum swing to patient autonomy; autonomy in itself appears not to be the answer. When the medical dialogue is a shared process, outcomes appear to be better. Neither physician dominance nor total abdication of power are related to positive patient outcomes; rather, engagement in a process that leads to agreement on problem and problem solving appears to be the optimum alternative.

The psychological mechanisms by which patients gain these health benefits can be unclear and several alternatives are possible. First, improved communication may produce more satisfaction, which in turn produces more confidence in the doctor, which in turn maximizes nonspecific healing mechanisms; these patients may attribute more positive motives to their caretakers, viewing them as supportive, concerned, understanding, and reassuring. Furthermore, patients who faithfully follow through with medical recommendations maximize the therapeutic benefit from their regimens and make health care more effective. Indeed, a meta-analysis showed that better adherence predicted better health outcomes, especially for chronic diseases (DiMatteo, Giordani, Lepper, & Croghan, 2002).

But other mechanisms by which communication enhances patient health are also possible. Some kinds of communication may affect patients' health status by increasing self-confidence and motivation. Patients who perceive themselves as capable of affecting their own health in a positive manner may act healthier, and in fact become healthier, than those with poor health self-concepts and a lack of confidence in their own abilities. Moreover, an increased sense of participation in medical care decisions through more active, two-way communication may be linked with a positive perception of mastery and control over one's total environment, including health, leading to a more self-confident and powerful life outlook. We discuss several intervention studies in the next chapter that have experimentally linked enhanced communication with better clinical outcomes.

PHYSICIAN OUTCOMES

Satisfied physicians are more likely to have satisfied patients, and doctors who enjoy their work are more likely to be better at it—or at least happier while doing it than dissatisfied physicians. However, not all physicians are equally satisfied or well suited for their career. Estimates are that, although most physicians report being satisfied (40%) or very satisfied (40%), one in five physicians is dissatisfied (Leigh, Kravitz, Schembri, Samuels, & Mobley, 2002). Contributors to career satisfaction vary widely, with some of these relating to the specialty in which the physician practices or to contextual and environmental aspects of practice, and others to physicians' personality and sociodemographic profile, and still others to the kinds of patients that the physician treats.

Based on reports from more than 12,000 physicians, Leigh and colleagues ranked respondents' assessments of career satisfaction and dissatisfaction across 33 specialty categories. Interestingly, the investigators note that not only were there obvious differences in satisfaction ratings between specialties but also physicians' responses within a given specialty varied. For example, orthopedic surgeons were both more satisfied and more dissatisfied than other doctors, suggesting a sharply divided workforce, while physical medicine and rehabilitation physicians were less satisfied and less dissatisfied than other physicians, suggesting fewer physicians with extreme sentiments among this group.

The five highest relative satisfaction ratings belonged to geriatric internal medicine, neonatal-perinatal medicine, dermatology, pediatrics, and "all other" specialties, while the highest percentages in the dissatisfied category belonged to otolaryngology, obstetrics-gynecology, ophthalmology, orthopedic surgery, and internal medicine. While a number of these ratings were as predicted, for instance high levels of satisfaction for dermatology and low levels for obstetrics-gynecology, others presented a surprise. The relatively high proportion of dissatisfied physicians among those in "procedural" specialties (i.e., ophthalmology, pulmonary medicine, orthopedic surgery, otolaryngology) was unexpected given the historically high income and prestige associated with them. The authors credit the relative loss in income and autonomy due to managed care and Medicare payment reform over the past 15 years for the poor ratings.

The authors also found that career satisfaction varied by a variety of environmental and sociodemographic characteristics. Physicians most likely to be very satisfied were at the beginning or end of their careers (younger than 35 or 65 and older), suggesting that the enthusiasm, and perhaps idealism, that is high when physicians first enter practice wanes considerably as they move through their career. Retirement for those who are least happy would explain the highly satisfied ratings of those physicians who continue in practice long after their colleagues have left. Satisfied physicians earn a good living and live well; they are likely to be board certified, to earn in excess of $250,000 a year, and to reside in towns or rural areas or in New England or the northwest central states.

Predictably, dissatisfied physicians work longer hours and make less money than others. It is also evident that foreign medical school graduates are disproportionately represented among the dissatisfied group. No doubt, the combination of cultural stresses, perceived and actual discrimination from patients and medical institutions, and the special demands of working in medically underserved areas contribute to these ratings. Dissatisfied physicians are also more engaged with managed care and reimbursement bureaucracies than others and are likely to be full or partial owners of a practice and receive a high percentage of their revenue through Medicaid, Medicare, or managed care.

Relatively few studies of physician satisfaction have investigated how the doctor-patient relationship may contribute to physicians' positive feelings toward their medical work. Nevertheless, there is evidence that the physicians' rating of interpersonal rapport with patients, the personality demands of patients, as well as their ability to efficiently elicit a medical history from a patient and effectively use visit time are all thought to be important contributing factors to whether a physician feels that a particular visit was satisfying (Suchman, Roter, Greene, & Lipkin, 1993). Two of these satisfaction dimensions, effective use of time and efficient data gathering, tend to be stable for individual physicians across a range of patients whereas satisfaction with the patient-physician relationship and personality demands are variable, and consequently, unique to each patient (Suchman et al., 1993).

The nature of medical visit communication was also found to predict physician satisfaction. Physicians were less satisfied, particularly with the use of visit time and adequacy of data collection, in visits in which they were verbally dominant and focused on biomedical questions and explanations of medical symptoms and treatment. In contrast, visits that can be considered patient centered, by the inclusion of even modest levels of psychosocial, emotional, and partnership exchanges with patients, were viewed by physicians as especially satisfying (Roter et al., 1997). In a similar vein, the physicians reported less success at accomplishing visit goals in narrowly biomedical visits than in the more psychosocially inclusive visits.

As noted earlier in this chapter, a patient's health status is related to the patient's satisfaction. It is also true that physicians are more satisfied in visits with healthier patients (J. A. Hall et al., 1993; J. A. Hall et al., 2002). This finding may contribute to an understanding of the special case of burnout among oncologists. As many as one-third of oncologists suffer emotional exhaustion and a sense of low personal accomplishment, with as many as one-quarter having a psychiatric disorder (Ramirez, Graham, Richards, Cull, & Gregory, 1996). The problem appears to be getting worse. A recent follow-up on the earlier study found that the prevalence of psychiatric morbidity has increased to fully one-third of surveyed clinical and surgical oncologists, with as many as 40% reporting emotional exhaustion (Cath, Graham, Potts, Richards, & Ramirez, 2005).

Extraordinary expectations may contribute to the stress burden these oncologists carry; they are expected to be scientifically expert providers who are both technologically competent and empathic communicators, able to deal with patients' physical and psychological distress, and able to respond to distressed, angry, and blaming relatives (Cath et al., 2005). Dealing with patients' emotional reactions to cancer has emerged as one of the primary areas of communication difficulty for senior cancer clinicians attending training courses in England (Ford, Fallowfield, & Lewis, 1996). Lacking formal training in this area, many of these doctors develop cold, detached styles of communication. Though detachment may provide some emotional protection, it appears more illusory than real. It is the emotional connection with patients that allows doctors to establish the sort of therapeutic relationship that is a source of satisfaction for oncologists (Fallowfield, 1995). It is telling that the only positive area of their work in which oncologists reported increased job satisfaction was in relationships with patients, relatives, and staff (Cath et al., 2005).

MALPRACTICE

At its extreme, low satisfaction can contribute to a negative spiraling of confidence and regard, sometimes culminating in a malpractice litigation. Research finds that disappointment in one's relationship with a physician often overshadows the objective severity of the physician's errors of medical judgment. Objectively measured quality of care does not appear to be the primary determinant in a patient's decision to initiate a malpractice claim. It is estimated that fewer than 2% of patients who have actually suffered a significant injury due to negligence initiate a malpractice claim (Localio, Lawthers, & Brennan, 1991). Many experts would argue that the malpractice crisis facing the country is not caused by compensation of patients who have been harmed but rather by litigation from patients who have been disappointed or offended by some aspect of the physician's interpersonal manner. It is the addition of insult, in the form of perceived uncaring or indifference, to injury that is often cited as the deciding factor for patients in pursuing legal remedy. In either case, it appears that patients and families are more likely to sue a physician when faced with a bad outcome if they felt that the physician failed to communicate in a timely and open manner (Beckman, Markakis, Suchman, & Frankel, 1994).

Whether sued physicians actually communicate differently than other physicians was explored in a study by Levinson, Roter, Mullooly, Dull, and Frankel (1997). This study was designed to investigate whether routine medical visit communication was related, either as a result or a cause, to the malpractice claim experience of surgeons or primary care physicians. Malpractice claims in this study were defined as any patient request for funds, any malpractice suit filed by a patient, or any contact by an attorney who represented a patient in an action against the physician, regardless of outcome.

The study was quite large and included over 1,200 patient visits with 65 surgeons and 59 primary care doctors. The doctors were matched based on their specialties and number of years in practice, but half of the physicians had never been sued and the other half had two or more lifetime malpractice claims. Researchers were sent to each doctor's office, and 10 random patients were audiotape recorded during a routine visit. Interaction analysis of the physician visits (using the RIAS coding system described in Chapter 3) found that there were a number of differences in the way the sued and nonsued physicians talked with their patients. Eighty percent of primary care physicians were accurately classified in terms of malpractice status based on their communication patterns—a 30% improvement over chance. The sued doctors had shorter visits, by almost three minutes, used less partnership-type exchanges (i.e., asking for the patient's opinion, understanding of what was said, and expectations for the visit; showing interest in patient disclosures; and paraphrasing and interpreting what the patient said), engaged in less humor and laughter, and were less likely to orient the patient to what to expect in regard to the flow of the visit than physicians who had never been sued.

The communication analysis did not work quite as well for surgeons as it did for primary care physicians. While none of the communication elements was a statistically significant predictor of the surgeons' malpractice status, several variables showed a similar trend. Sued surgeons had shorter visits, by almost 1.5 minutes, and used less partnership-type exchanges. Interestingly, some variables appeared to go in the opposite direction than what would be expected based on the primary care findings. For instance, there was significantly *more* patient laughter in the surgical visits of sued doctors compared to those who were not sued, but no difference in physician laughter in these visits. Why might this be so? While laughter is usually associated with positive affect and a relaxed and friendly atmosphere, it can also reflect something quite different—an indication of nervousness, embarrassment, or anxiety (Sala, Krupat, & Roter, 2002). We do not know for sure if the quality of laughter differed in these visits, but it is possible that the relatively high levels of patient laughter suggests that there may be more tension in these visits than in those of nonclaims surgeons.

To further investigate the emotional tone of the surgical visits, a thin-slice analysis of the surgeons' interactions was conducted (Ambady et al., 2002). Thin-slice analysis relies on very short segments of speech or video clips, as short as a few seconds. In this case, the speech segments were stripped of literal content by an electronic filter and judged by multiple raters on a variety of affective dimensions (including concern/anxiety and dominance). Two patients were chosen for each of the study's 65 surgeons (the most satisfied and the most dissatisfied) and a 10-second speech segment was taken from the first and last minute of the visits. Surgeons judged to have more dominant voice tone were almost three times as likely to be in the sued group than others, while the surgeons whose voice tone was rated as conveying concern/anxiety were half as likely to be in the sued group.

We hypothesize that the patients interpret dominant voice tones differently than anxious voice tones. On the one hand, dominance communicates an imperious or overbearing manner, or perhaps a lack of empathy and understanding, or even indifference. Anxiety in the physician's voice tone, on the other hand, may be heard as seriousness, attentiveness, and concern for the patient's well-being and future health. Our earlier studies using thin-slice analysis found that anxious voice tone coupled with positive words (sympathetic and calming) was associated with more patient satisfaction and better appointment keeping over a 6-month period (J. A. Hall et al., 1981). In this context, we think that voice tone may act to frame the way in which the verbal message is interpreted. A second study similarly linked anxious vocal qualities with patient satisfaction (Roter et al., 1987).

Going back to the malpractice study, we can suggest that the nonsued doctors sounded less overbearing and more conscientious and attentive—qualities that patients find desirable in a physician. The interpretation of the study results, however, is not completely straightforward. The study could not answer the question of whether the communication style and voice tone characteristics were associated with a heightened risk of being sued, or whether the experience of being sued changed how the doctors felt about, or communicated with, their patients. There is support for both explanations, and perhaps both are true.

It is clear that physicians differ in their communication styles and orientations toward patients, and these factors are related to their patients' satisfaction, confidence, and trust. Moreover, it has been argued that these characteristics can act to protect a physician from, or put a physician at risk for, litigation, should an adverse event occur. Once a physician is sued, however, there is reason to believe that the experience itself is transforming. Malpractice litigation can be a demoralizing, even traumatizing, event for a physician. The physician may feel and act angry and defensive after being sued, and, consequently, perhaps raise his or her risk of even more complaints and suits (Hickson et al., 2002). In commenting on the transforming effect of a malpractice suit on colleagues, Dr. Abraham Verghese, a physician and novelist who has written on the subject, noted in a *New York Times* article that after coming through a long malpractice suit, a physician friend of his had said, "Now I think of the patient as the enemy" (Verghese, 2003, p. 11). As discussed earlier in this chapter, liking matters in relationships; patients search for cues by which to judge their relationships with their doctors—they look to see if the physicians care about them and will go the extra mile for them. Verghese goes on to say, "A wise former judge once told me, 'Patients who like their doctors don't sue, no matter what their lawyer says.' Our efforts in medical schools to turn out skilled yet empathic physicians who communicate clearly and who can put themselves in their patients' shoes are critical to stemming the malpractice crisis. Patients sue when their feelings are ignored or when they are angered by lack of genuine concern for their welfare. . . . Though it provides no guarantee, a sound physician-patient relationship is a powerful antidote to frivolous lawsuits" (p. 12).

Relationships matter to both patients and physicians and the relationship itself may be the most powerful antidote to the malpractice crisis that medicine can provide.

10

Improving Talk through Interventions

Imagine you are a man in your fifties, suffering a long 2 days in the hospital before your coronary bypass surgery. You have many questions about what's about to happen, and naturally you have fears too. Your hospital roommate is also awaiting surgery, but his surgery is to fuse the vertebrae in his back following a long history of disc trouble.

Suppose you are an 80-year-old woman living in a nursing home. You can get around with your walker, but you often wonder what the point is—you seem to be losing some of your interest in things. One day the director, speaking to you and others living on your floor, reminds you that you have responsibility for this as your home and should decide how you want your room to look.

Now, imagine you are a man of 75, quite alert and energetic, but burdened with a growing list of ailments for which you regularly see your doctor. Sometimes you get confused about the increasingly complex explanations and drug regimens your doctor offers. In fact, last time your daughter asked about your health, you found you didn't have the answers to several obviously important questions and had to admit you were not sure you were taking all the drugs you were supposed to.

How wonderful it would be if one could decrease the anxiety of the man in the hospital, increase the zest of the woman in the nursing home, and improve the elderly man's understanding of his regimen. Is it at all possible? What is the cost? How elaborate or intense an effort would have to be made by someone—a doctor, social worker, psychologist, family member, administrator—to achieve these gains? Has anyone tried?

Throughout this book, we have asserted our conviction that doctors and patients can change their interactions for the better, and we have spent most of these pages arguing that change is needed and theoretically possible. Now we intend to show that talk between doctors and patients (and, in one study, between patients) has been shown to be both cause and consequence of many important features of medical care.

We have been careful about using such terms as cause and consequence, for much of the available research is not designed to ascertain with confidence what, if anything, caused a change to occur (for example, what causes the state of one's health or how satisfied one is with care). Frequently, a researcher knows that two variables are associated but is not at all sure that one is responsible for the other. However, in controlled experiments or, to use an alternative term, randomized controlled trials, one gains such confidence because, in these studies, the researcher determines who will and who will not receive different experimental treatments (also called interventions) and administers them to groups of people who are otherwise equivalent. An experiment is designed so that only the special treatment or the intervention could be responsible for subsequent changes in health or behavior.

Numerous experiments have demonstrated that talk can be changed and that talk can have powerful effects in the medical visit. It can also be surprisingly simple and inexpensive to engineer these changes. This is an extremely important point. If beneficial changes come only with major attitudinal overhauls, extensive training or education, lots of extra attention from research or clinical personnel, or expensive reorganization of the structure of care, then the chances of such interventions ever finding their way into everyday attitudes, medical education, and routine clinical practice are slight, or at least a long way off.

The interventions we plan to tell you about addressed common and everyday problems of patients and physicians, were all relatively straightforward and simple, and yet had impressive results.

PREPAREDNESS, INFORMATION, AND HEALTH

In the actual research from which we extracted the hypothetical gentleman awaiting surgery mentioned earlier, some coronary bypass patients were assigned to semiprivate rooms in which their roommates had not yet undergone surgery (as in the example), whereas others were assigned to semiprivate rooms whose other occupants had already had their operations (Kulik & Mahler, 1987; Kulik, Moore, & Mahler, 1993; Kulik, Mahler, & Moore, 1996). If the roommate was postoperative, the patient awaiting surgery was significantly less anxious prior to surgery, according to a combined measure of self-rated anxiety, nurse-rated anxiety, and number of tranquilizing medications taken in the 2 days before surgery. Remarkably, the beneficial effects did not end there. These patients walked more in the first 3 days after surgery and left the hospital a full 1.4 days sooner than patients whose roommates before surgery were also preoperative.

How could such a simple thing as roommate assignment make such a difference? The answer is that under conditions of uncertainty, people look around for cues as to how to react and feel, emotionally and physically. In this study, patients must have looked to their roommates for clues as to how anxious to feel. Because the postoperative roommates were undoubtedly less anxious than they had been before the operation, the patients awaiting surgery were less anxious too. These patients probably gained relief from knowledge that the roommates had survived and seemed generally in one piece. The patients may also have learned from their postoperative roommates particular kinds of information that helped them prepare for the experience—what exactly happened, what it felt like, and so forth (Kulik & Mahler, 1987).

Indeed, a wealth of research demonstrates the beneficial effects of preparedness on coping and recovery. This preparedness comes from both factual knowledge about one's medical condition and about what to expect, and from reassurance and support provided by care providers or others at crucial points in the process. One mechanism whereby information produces positive health effects is the enhanced sense of control that comes when one is able to predict what will happen. Feeling in control of events and circumstances has wide-ranging effects in both the health domain and in other aspects of everyday life. People who feel they have control can better tolerate pain and bodily symptoms. They report fewer health problems, have better health status, and recover more quickly from illness.

A landmark study by Egbert and associates in the 1960s began a revolution in patient preparation for surgical procedures (Egbert, Battit, Welch, & Bartlett, 1964). In this study, a physician spent about 20 minutes with a patient the evening before surgery to talk about postoperative pain and self-care exercises that might speed the recovery process. The simple intervention resulted in use of half the usual pain medication and discharge from the hospital almost 3 days earlier than control patients. Far from unique, this first study has been replicated and extended to a great number and variety of clinical conditions in which the provision of information or psychological preparation to patients led to positive clinical outcomes (Mumford, Schlesinger, & Glass, 1982; Devine 1992). By 1992, 191 studies tested the effects of providing health care relevant information, self-care exercises, and psychosocial support (broadly referred to as psychoeducational interventions) on a variety of patient outcomes, including recovery from surgery, reductions in length of hospital stay, pain control, and emotional distress.

Depending on the outcome studied, the percentage of studies indicating beneficial effects ranged from 79% to 84% (Devine, 1992).

The interventions covered a range of activities performed by psychiatrists, psychologists, surgeons, anesthesiologists, nurses, and others. Sometimes the programs were elaborate, but often they were simple and inexpensive modifications of standard medical procedures. A typical study of this kind invited male preoperative patients to meet in a small group led by a nurse the evening before surgery. The participants discussed concerns and fears about the surgery and also heard about what to expect and how to aid in their own recuperation. Compared to comparable control group patients who underwent similar surgery, the experimental group patients slept better, were less anxious the morning of surgery, required less anesthesia and pain medication, suffered less postoperative urinary retention, returned more rapidly to oral intake, and were discharged sooner from the hospital (Schmitt & Woolridge, 1973).

In some studies in this area, the preparedness intervention was not even with the patient (children undergoing tonsillectomy and adenoidectomy), but was rather with the patient's parent (Mahaffy, 1965). In this case, the intervention had dramatic effects, even when filtered through the patients' mothers. The mothers received two brief sessions designed to provide information and support from a nurse. The first session was upon admission to the hospital and the second when the child returned from the recovery room. Children of mothers receiving the intervention were better able to drink liquids, had less vomiting, and cried less during the hospital stay. A follow-up questionnaire completed at home by each child's mother also found much better outcomes for the intervention group. Children of prepared mothers were reported to have had less fever, less disturbed sleep, and less fear of doctors and nurses. The mothers also reported fewer doctor visits to the home during the recovery period. We can speculate that a mother who is informed and whose anxieties are relieved will explain things better and will behave in a more relaxed and optimistic way, conveying to her child that things are going fine, that it's not so scary, and that she's not worried.

The positive effects of providing information to patients as a means of reducing stress outside the hospital setting have also been demonstrated (Fuller, Endress, & Johnson, 1978; Johnson & Leventhal, 1974; Johnson, Kirchoff, & Endress, 1975). The bulk of these studies assessed the effect of information and preparedness as a means of reducing stress related to unpleasant medical examinations (such as endoscopy, removal of orthopedic casts, or pelvic exams) and demonstrate the wide potential use of information techniques in office settings.

Despite evidence of the substantial benefit of the psychoeducation programs described above, implementation of these programs—both inside and outside of hospital settings—tends to be haphazard and far less than optimal.

As a consequence, many patients who could benefit from these simple interventions fail to have the opportunity to do so (Devine, 1992; Mullen, van den Borne, & Breemhaar, 2000; Kain & Caldwell-Andrews, 2005).

EMPOWERING PATIENTS TO BE ACTIVELY ENGAGED IN THEIR HEALTH

Now we turn to the woman we introduced earlier, who lives in a nursing home. The nursing home administrator told her and her floormates not only that they should decide on the appearance of their rooms, but that they should decide on many details of their daily lives, such as when and whom to visit on the floor, when to watch television, and which movies they would like. He invited them to suggest changes to the staff, and then offered each of them a houseplant that would be the patient's responsibility.

In this well-known research, the nursing home patients were followed for over a year, as were those on a different floor who were addressed by their administrator but not reminded of the various choices they could make nor of the need to take responsibility for themselves (Langer & Rodin, 1976; Rodin & Langer, 1977). Rather, he emphasized that it was the nursing home's responsibility to keep them happy and well cared for. He covered all the same topics, and he gave them a plant, but he did not focus on choice and responsibility.

The results of this study were as dramatic as the intervention was subtle. Patients in the responsibility-induced group were later happier, more active, more alert, and more improved in health; they spent more time talking with staff and fellow patients; and they had a death rate of 15% in the 18 months following the intervention, compared to a death rate of 30% in the comparison group. There can be no doubt that a large share of these effects stemmed from processes internal to the patients that were triggered by the administrator's message. People's capacities are influenced by what they expect those capacities to be. The "will to live" is now a confirmed notion in medicine. In addition, the responsibility-induced patients who now talked more to staff and to other patients were probably pleased with the positive effect their interactions had on others' attitudes toward them, which further enhanced self-esteem and the sense of meaningful belonging to a group. Moreover, talking more to medical or nursing staff surely must have had effects on the process of medical care. As noted in previous chapters, patients who are happier and healthier are likely to engage in more positive and satisfying communication with their physicians and other care givers, perhaps receiving more positive regard, social support, attention, and the confidence to engage in other self-care behaviors in a confident and active manner.

Earlier, in Chapter 8, we described how important information is but noted that patients ask few questions and seldom make forceful demands for information from their physician. Some reasons for such reticence include lack of forethought and preparation for the visit, and the skill to clearly articulate ideas or questions. Perhaps, then, patients need help in developing their question-asking skills. Just such a study was first conducted in 1977 (Roter, 1977). Half the patients attending a community health clinic were randomly assigned to an experiment to increase the number of questions they asked during their medical visit while the other half of the patients were given a session on a topic unrelated to question asking. This was a simple intervention that took about 10 minutes in the waiting room prior to the patient's visit with the doctor.

The health educator, together with the patient, worked through a question-asking protocol to identify questions the patient may have had about his or her illness or treatment. The protocol was structured to review possible questions in the areas of disease etiology, symptom duration, severity of illness, prevention and lifestyle-related suggestions, and treatment, including medications, diet, and physical therapy. If the patient indicated that he or she had no questions in a particular area, the educator would proceed to the next area. After covering the entire protocol the educator would read back the list of questions and close the session by assuring the patient that the questions identified were important and encouraging the patient to actually ask the questions of the doctor.

This process did not produce long lists of questions; patients receiving the intervention asked on average slightly less than two questions when they were with their doctors. However, this was enough to produce changes in the way patients viewed themselves and in the communication process. As part of the study, patients' locus of control was measured. This is a measure that reflects the tendency for individuals to see themselves as powerless in the face of destiny, luck, or other people, versus powerful in the sense of controlling their own good or bad fortune. The sense of control is subject to change based on experience, and patients who participated in the intervention underwent such a change in attitude and self-image. They felt more in control and responsible for their health, and they acted on these feelings by being more active in the medical visit and asking more questions. Analysis of tape recordings of the visits found that the number of questions patients asked during the medical visit doubled for those participating in the intervention compared to a control group. Moreover, over the next 6 months, intervention group patients more consistently kept appointments with their doctors than those in the control group.

By 2004, a systematic review of intervention studies designed to increase patient participation during the medical visit identified 20 such studies

(Harrington, Noble, & Newman, 2004). Though the interventions varied, the majority targeted question asking as the primary mechanism of activating patients to be more engaged in the medical dialogue. The format of interventions included face to face coaching, as in the earliest study, but also print aids such as booklets and checklists, and multimedia approaches that modeled question asking behavior. The authors concluded that, overall, the interventions had a significant effect in helping patients to be more active in their visits. Most interventions were successful in increasing the number of questions asked or concerns raised with the coaching and video interventions being especially successful. At least some of the studies, although not all, compared the intervention to usual care or to a comparison intervention designed to mimic the amount of attention and time of the intervention but not the activation emphasis. Consequently, it is unlikely that the positive results are simply an attention or placebo effect.

Some of these studies went further in their analysis than simply demonstrating greater patient activity in the visit and explored the impact of a more active patient role on health outcomes. Among the first of the studies to address health impact was one conducted by Greenfield and colleagues (Greenfield, Kaplan, & Ware, 1985; Greenfield, Kaplan, Ware, Yano, & Frank, 1988; Kaplan, Greenfield, & Ware, 1989). These researchers designed an intervention that was tested first with a group of patients with peptic ulcer disease and then replicated in patients with hypertension, diabetes, and cancer. During the 20 minutes immediately preceding the medical visit, half the patients were approached by a clinic assistant who, together with each patient, reviewed the patient's medical record, acquainted the patient with treatment protocols for his or her condition, and encouraged the patient to ask questions about his or her care and discuss treatment decisions with his or her doctor. The investigators then tape-recorded the visit and gathered postvisit questionnaires from patients and doctors, including a mailed questionnaire nearly 2 months later.

Analysis of study audiotapes showed that the activated patients were significantly more active in the conversation with the doctor, were much more assertive, and elicited twice the number of factual statements from the doctor. Activated patients also reported significantly fewer physical limitations in the weeks that followed the visit, and less limitation on their ability to work and perform other important social roles. The more active they were in the visit (talking more, asking more questions, being more assertive), the better was their reported health later. And the patients seemed to like this new role, for they expressed a significantly stronger preference for active involvement in medical decision making. The hypertensive patients receiving the activation intervention had improved quality of life and functional status ratings, as well as lowered blood pressure measured during the follow-up period. Diabetic patients demonstrated all the same positive effects, as well as lowered blood glucose upon follow-up, indicating better control of their diabetic condition. The experience of breast cancer patients also paralleled the others. In this case, symptom experience was monitored through patients' diaries and was found to lessen for intervention group patients over the course of chemotherapy.

Several explanations of possible mechanisms by which these health changes were accomplished can be suggested. Inasmuch as more patient control, more engagement (marked especially by negative affect, expressed by both patients and physicians), and more information provided by physicians during office visits were associated with better subsequent health status, the authors suggested that these aspects of communication reflect "healthy friction" or role tension between physicians and patients (Kaplan et al., 1989). Patients' assertions of control through more effective information seeking, and perhaps disagreements, transform an otherwise physician-dominated monologue into a two-way exchange in which the patient has an active role and an obvious stake. The patient thus engaged is invested, perhaps more than otherwise, in the process as well as the outcome of the visit. It is also possible that negative expressions of frustration by the physician with a patient who is not progressing as expected may be interpreted by the patient as an expression of caring on the part of the physician.

In our own work, we have found that when physicians sound angry and anxious, their patients are more satisfied and compliant. We believe that they attribute more concern and sincerity to a physician who is emotionally engaged than to one who appears emotionally neutral (J. A. Hall, Roter, & Rand, 1981).The talk of the medical visit has an influence on patients' health status over and above its specific contribution to diagnosis and therapeutic activities. We agree with Kaplan and colleagues that the physician-patient relationship is a primary bond that may act as a form of social support to influence patients' health status (Kaplan et al., 1989).

Because of the magnitude of positive results, and because the researchers were successful in replicating their intervention in separate clinical trials conducted with patients of different socioeconomic and ethnic backgrounds and medical conditions, the findings are especially important. Attempts by other investigators to replicate the intervention, however, have met with mostly disappointing results (Griffin et al., 2004). It is not hard to think of how people—both patients and doctors—from southern Californian differ from others in ways that may account for their greater responsivity to activation interventions. Regardless, this series of studies has been instrumental in investigating the health effects of communication interventions.

To help readers get a better sense of the activation protocols used in the studies reviewed above, we have included a guide to asking questions

(Table 10.1). It is based on our own past work and the work of others, notably David Tuckett and his colleagues in England (Tuckett, Boulton, Olson, & Williams, 1985).

USE OF MEDICAL RECORDS

Another way to engage patients in their care is to give them access to their medical record (S. E. Ross & Lin, 2003). This would have been helpful to the elderly gentleman, mentioned in our opening vignette, who was unsure of important facts regarding his health and medical regimen. This simple intervention appears to produce benefits. For instance, in one study investigators simply mailed elderly patients copies of their physicians' progress notes from the most recent visit (typewritten for legibility), and discovered that patients gained greater understanding of their health problems and their treatments, compared to a group of similar patients in a control group (Bronson, Costanza, & Tufo, 1986).

Other studies have found that the provision of the medical record to pregnant women is an especially effective way of enhancing communication, increasing a sense of control, and optimizing involvement in decision making during prenatal care (Brown & Smith, 2004). A good example of these type benefits is found in a study in which women who were randomized to receive a complete copy of their medical record through their pregnancy were compared to those who received an abbreviated information card (the standard practice) (Homer, Davis, & Everitt, 1999). The women with full records were significantly more likely to report feeling "in control" during pregnancy whereas the other women reported feeling more anxious and helpless about their pregnancy and its outcome. Moreover, women who received their records reported greater ease in talking with their health care providers and had more information on their records explained to them (Homer et al., 1999). Not only were women better informed, but their partners were too. The women who were given their records reported using them to share information with their partners, especially when their partners could not attend their appointments with them.

It is especially noteworthy that a common theme in malpractice depositions and complaints lodged against obstetricians is poor communication, including the feeling that their physicians would not talk to them or answer questions, listen to their concerns, or inform them of their infants' medical conditions during or after labor and delivery (Hickson, Clayton, Githens, & Sloan, 1992). Perhaps providing a medical record would have improved communication in these instances and alleviated some of the terrible distress suffered by these families and their physicians.

Table 10.1
A Patient's Guide to Asking Questions

Asking questions is a very important part of your visit to the doctor. By asking questions, your doctor can help clear up doubts, concerns, or worries. It is an important way in which you can get things straight. Don't just worry about something, ask!!

A. Diagnosis	Has the doctor told you what the nature of your problem is? That is, has the doctor told you what the diagnosis is? Do you think the diagnosis is correct, or that something else or something more is the problem?
B. Etiology	Do you know what caused your problem?
C. Prognosis	Have you discussed the seriousness of this problem with the doctor? Do you know how long your problem will last? Do you know how long it will be until there is an improvement? Are you worried that it will come back or get worse? Are you worried about how this problem may be affecting your health in the long run?
D. Treatment	Do you know how the doctor proposes to treat your problem? Do you understand why the doctor thinks this treatment is the best? Is there any other kind of treatment that you think might work?
E. Medications	Has your doctor prescribed any medication for you? If so: Do you know the name of the medication? Do you know how the medication helps you? Do you know when to take the medication? For instance, do you know what to do if you miss a dose? Should you take two doses when you remember, or should you just skip the missed dose? If the drug is prescribed every 4 hours, does that mean you should waken during the night to take your dose? Do you know what possible side effects are associated with the medicine? For example, is it likely to make you drowsy or nauseated? Is the drug likely to interact with alcohol or with any over-the-counter, nonprescription drugs you may be taking?
F. Tests	Has your doctor ordered any tests? If so, are you sure of the purpose of the tests that have been ordered and what the results will be used for?
G. Lifestyle	Has the doctor suggested a change in any lifestyle habits, such as smoking, drinking alcohol, exercise, weight, or diet? If so: Do you know how much change is needed to make a difference? Were you given any hints about how to make these changes easier?
H. Prevention	Do you know what you can do to prevent this problem in the future? Do you know if your problem "runs in the family"? If so, do you know what you can do to help others from developing this problem?

The experience of other groups of patients with medical records also appears to be positive. Williams and colleagues found that providing medical records to patients undergoing cancer treatment was helpful in preparing for appointments, reducing difficulties in monitoring their own progress, and helping them to feel more in control (J. G. Williams et al., 2001). In this study, however, only about half of the participants indicated that they preferred to keep their own records, while the others were indifferent to the suggestion. Younger patients with more professionals involved in their care seemed to benefit most from having their records and these patients were most likely to indicate a preference for continuing the practice.

It has been noted that the recent technological advances have increased the convenience and portability of electronic patient records making it far easier for patients to maintain a current copy of their medical record than ever before. These advances have also made the patient record more attractive as an educational and motivational tool for the advancement of a more collaborative partnership (S. E. Ross & Lin, 2003).

USE OF VISIT AUDIOTAPES

For some patients, a greater feeling of control may come with confidence that they have not misunderstood, forgotten, or invented information conveyed by their doctor during their medical visit. These type issues may be especially salient for patients with a negative prognosis. For instance, one study found that almost half the cancer patients questioned felt that the information the doctor gave to them at the "bad news" visit had been inadequate. Most of these patients acknowledged, however, that the diagnosis of cancer had so shocked or stunned them that they were unable to recall very much of the rest of the conversation (Fallowfield, Baum, & Maguire, 1986). For these patients, having an audio recording of a critical medical visit, for instance one in which a life-threatening diagnosis was given or complicated treatment options discussed, may constitute an effective informational intervention and an easily accessible reality check.

A number of researchers have explored the potential utility of audiotapes to patients in intervention studies. For instance, in an early study in the area, patients with a diagnosis of either bowel or breast cancer were invited to take the recording of their visit home with them along with a questionnaire assessing its usefulness (Hogbin & Fallowfield, 1989). Virtually all the patients reported listening to the tape and said that it was useful in several ways. Patients indicated that the tape was helpful in clarifying points of confusion and reminding them of forgotten information, that it served to reassure and calm them, and that the tape made it easier for them to convey the distressing information to family and friends. Some of the comments, as reported by patients on the questionnaires, are especially telling. One patient noted, "I found the tape very helpful indeed for the reasons below: (1) it prevented me from unintentionally distorting any information I was given; (2) the calm and factual discussion is very useful to listen to again at times of panic and despair." Another patient noted to the doctor, "Your idea of the tape was brilliant, as I found I couldn't tell my family. They found it very helpful and put their minds at rest. Your tape gave me great comfort and confidence in you" (Hogbin & Fallowfield, 1989, p. 332).

A dozen additional studies of this nature have been conducted since the 1980s, almost all of them directed toward cancer patients (Santo, Laizner, & Shohet, 2005). On the whole, patients accepted and valued the information provided by the audiotapes and cancer patients appeared to benefit with at least some of these studies showing decreases in anxiety, increases in informational recall, facilitated decision making, and increased satisfaction (Santo et al., 2005).

INTERVENTIONS WITH PHYSICIANS

It can be argued that physicians are a much more efficient target of interventions than patients. After all, an intervention that changes a single physician's behavior is likely to affect thousands of patients each year. While it has long been assumed that physicians inevitably develop whatever communication skill they may need naturally or through experience, medical educators now agree that training is necessary. Unfortunately, the reality is that physicians perform hundreds of thousands of medical interviews during their career, often with minimal formal instruction (Lipkin, Putnam, & Lazare, 1995).

At this point, a solid foundation of behavioral science research demonstrates that training improves the communication of physicians. Communication skills training during medical school has been shown to have effects lasting as long as 5 years (Maguire, Fairbairn, & Fletcher, 1989). If the change lasts that long, it is probably permanent. Despite variations in the length and format of physician training programs, all or most focus on the principles of relationship-centered medicine as defined in this book (e.g., Bensing & Sluijs, 1985; Cohen-Cole, 1991; Novack, Dube, & Goldstein, 1992; Putnam, Stiles, Jacob, & James, 1988; Roter et al., 1995; Smith et al., 2000). Some illustrative training programs and their outcomes are described below.

Inui and associates developed a brief training program for doctors to improve the compliance of patients with high blood pressure (Inui, Yourtee, & Williamson, 1976). The training included a one-time teaching session (1 to 2 hours in length) given to internal medicine residents. During the session, findings from an earlier study were presented that documented widespread patient noncompliance with hypertension medications. Simple means for identifying the noncompliant patient were emphasized. The session also emphasized the need for physicians to include an analysis of the patient's knowledge, attitudes, and beliefs regarding his or her medical problems as part of the patient's history and physical exam. In fact, the study's approach required that the physicians learn a different doctoring role—one that de-emphasized the physician's job as a diagnostician and emphasized his or her role as a patient educator. Strategies for enhancing patient compliance were reviewed, including the relation of patients' ideas to their perception of the seriousness of hypertension, susceptibility to its complications, and the efficacy of therapy.

The results of the study were dramatic. Trained physicians allocated a greater percentage of clinic-visit time to patient education than did control physicians. This resulted in increased patient knowledge and more appropriate patient beliefs regarding hypertension and its therapy. Patients of the trained physicians were more compliant with drug regimens and had better control of blood pressure than control group patients. These changes were still evident 6 months after the tutorials.

An intervention was designed for pediatricians with the goal of enhancing patient (mother/child) compliance with antibiotic regimens (Maiman, Becker, Liptak, Nazarian, & Rounds, 1988). Ninety-one physicians were randomly assigned to one of three groups; two of these were treatment groups and the third a control group. The first group received a two-session tutorial, totaling 5 hours, as well as supplemental reading material on pediatric compliance with drug regimens. The tutorial sessions addressed the magnitude and determinants of noncompliance and provided practical compliance-enhancing strategies including the use of supplemental written instructions, simplifying dosage and scheduling of drugs when possible, and stressing ways to monitor compliance.

To compare the usefulness of the tutorial with a less expensive alternative, the second group of physicians did not attend the tutorial but received, through the mail, the same reading materials on patient compliance made available to the first group. Over a 6-month period following the intervention, mothers of children with otitis media who were given a 10-day antibiotic regimen were randomly selected by the research staff from the participating pediatricians' appointment rosters. Within 8 days of the medical visit, a home interview was conducted in which the mothers were questioned about their doctor's communication behavior during the medical visit. Mothers were also asked about the extent to which they adhered to the full 10-day drug regimen.

Both groups of intervention doctors performed much better than physicians in the control group, but, surprisingly, there were few consistent differences between physicians in the two treatment interventions. Doctors attending the tutorials used more of the compliance-enhancing strategies than physicians receiving the printed materials, but the differences were not very great. Moreover, mothers of children seeing pediatricians in either of the trained groups were found to comply much better with prescribed antibiotic regimens than patients of control group physicians. Furthermore, these effects appeared to be longlasting. Patients who enrolled late in the study, that is up to 6 months after the physicians received the tutorials or mailed materials, showed the same positive effects as patients followed early in the study period.

A very different kind of training study targeting skills reflecting emotional self-awareness and sensitivity to patients was conducted by a group of Israeli investigators (Kramer, Ber, & Moore, 1987). In this study, Israeli medical students and their physician mentors participated in 10 90-minute sessions on interviewing skills held twice a week for 5 weeks. At these meetings the students talked about admitting a patient to the hospital, diagnosing a life-threatening disease, death and dying, teamwork, uncertainty, and chronic disease. In addition, time was taken for role playing, with the students and mentors playing the roles of patients, physicians, and family members. The students' and physicians' "rejecting behavior" was studied both before and after in visits with real patients. Rejecting behavior included sarcasm, contempt, verbal rejection, nonresponsiveness to the patient's statements, and evading eye contact.

The results were fascinating. First, it was evident that before training the medical students engaged in much less rejection than did the physicians. Students averaged about six negative behaviors per interview before training, while physicians averaged almost twice as many. One year after training, students engaged in an average of two rejection behaviors compared to the physicians' five. A control group of students who did not receive training averaged 11 rejecting behaviors. Thus, negativity was substantially lower for both medical students and physicians, even after a year, while members of the control group increased rejecting behaviors over time.

This study underscores the damage that physicians can do as role models to their students, and what the natural toll of increasing responsibility may be on medical students over time. Medical students imitate their clinical teachers' patterns of dealing with patients. If the teachers exhibit a dehumanized and rejecting pattern of communication with patients, the students learn that pattern. On a positive note, it is clear that the damage done to the young medical students' ability and inclination to be compassionate and empathic can be prevented, diminished, or undone. Further, it is reassuring to see that even well respected and established physicians can change longstanding patterns of communication for the better.

Just as treating patients in a rejecting manner is hurtful to the patient, so is the lack of empathic behaviors. But again, studies show that empathy can be improved in both medical students and experienced doctors (Fine & Therrien, 1977; Kalisch, 1971). For instance, doctors trained in empathy can improve their ability to indicate understanding and offer feelings, make eye contact, appear more attentive and interested, and encourage their patients to talk more.

The findings from these studies are quite encouraging in that many critics of interviewing skills training maintain that, though medical students' behavior may be amenable to change, physicians already practicing in the community have an entrenched interviewing style. This is not the case as reflected in the Israeli study just mentioned; nor is it the case in our own work. We designed a study to develop and evaluate a continuing medical education program for community-based, primary care physicians with the hope of improving their recognition and handling of patients' psychosocial problems (Roter et al., 1995). Sixty-nine doctors and 652 of their patients participated in the study. The study physicians were randomly assigned to one of two 8-hour experimental interviewing skills groups (emphasizing emotion handling or problem solving) or a nontreatment control group. The skills groups met twice, 1 week apart, for two 4-hour sessions during which most of the time was spent in small groups of three to five physicians, with a preceptor experienced in teaching interviewing skills and a simulated patient to assist in role playing. Table 10.2 displays key elements of the training curriculum.

The success of our teaching program was evaluated by going to the offices of all study physicians and tape recording them with a number of their actual patients. Because we were particularly interested in how the doctors dealt with emotionally distressed patients, we administered a standardized measure of patient distress, the General Health Questionnaire (GHQ), to all study patients. In this way we were able to tell which patients were likely to be suffering from mental distress and which were not, and we analyzed the audiotapes of an equal number of each type of patient. Each of the patients found to be distressed according to the screening questionnaire was called by telephone at 2 weeks, 3 months, and 6 months after the medical visit to assess the patient's health status—both physical and mental.

We found that the trained physicians did indeed use significantly more of the trained behaviors during the medical visits than control group physicians, and there were relatively few differences in performance between the two trained groups. We also found significant differences by treatment group in physicians' ability to identify patients in emotional distress. Trained physicians were better than control group physicians at recognizing which of their patients were distressed. Long-term effects of the intervention were also evident. Patients of trained doctors showed significantly greater improvement in their mental health than the control group patients up to 6 months following the medical visit.

Table 10.2
Critical Communication Skills for the Physician

I. Elicit the Full Spectrum of Patient Concerns

   (1) *Use open-ended questions*

      Example: What's been going on since I saw you last?

   (2) *Resist immediate follow-up*

      Example: I know you came in to have your mole checked. Is there anything else that is bothering you or causing you concern that you would like to discuss today?

   (3) *Set priorities by negotiating an agenda and use of time*

      Examples:

            —Of all these problems, which do you consider the most troubling?

            —There are a number of important things for us to work on. Which of these would you like to tackle today, and which could be taken up at our next visit?

II. Explore the Significance and Impact of the Problem

   (1) *Ask EXPLICITLY for the patient's opinion, experience, understanding, and interpretation*

      Examples:

            —What do you think your problem is?

            —Has anything like this happened before?

            —What do you think caused it?

            —What do you think it means?

            —What troubles you most about it?

   (2) *Ask EXPLICITLY for expectations*

      Example: What do you think I can do that would help?

III. Effectively Elicit and Respond to Patient Emotions

   (1) *Ask for feelings*

      Examples:

            —How do you feel about that?

            —What are your concerns?

            —Are you worried about anything related to this (condition)?

   (2) *Compliment patient effort*

      Example: I want you to know that I think you are doing a good job managing this complicated regimen.

Table 10.2
Critical Communication Skills for the Physician (Continued)

(3) *Legitimate the patient's feelings*

Example: I would be surprised if a person with your problem did not feel angry.

(4) *Express accurate empathy*

Verbal examples:

—You seem really anxious about this.

—You look worried (angry, anxious, hesitant, etc.).

Nonverbal examples:

—Lean your body forward; use a sad or sympathetic tone of voice; show a concerned or distressed facial expression.

—Physical contact (such as putting an arm around a patient's shoulder, squeezing a hand, or patting an arm) can enhance empathy, but should be used with care because patients show wide variation in their responses to uninvited physical contact.

As reflected in just the small sampling of patient and provider interventions reviewed in this chapter, we believe that there is tremendous potential to enhance the communication of medicine and optimize the therapeutic effect of those efforts.

Endnote

While there has been much fascinating work added to the literature in the years since the first edition of this book was written, we find that the key messages of our book have remained the same. There are three. First, we believe that the therapeutic potential of medicine can be enhanced—diagnoses made more accurate, treatments more effective, recoveries faster and less painful, and quality of life more fully realized. And, the vehicle by which this will be accomplished is the doctor-patient relationship.

Second, we believe that both doctors and patients can change the nature of their relationship and its interaction through modest interventions with far-reaching consequences. This is not to say that the determinants of behavior are simple. We have reviewed a great deal of research attesting to the complex nature of previous experience and culture on behavior; however, we are confident in our conclusion that the doctor-patient relationship is remarkably sensitive to change.

Finally, we believe that responsibility for change lies with both patients and physicians. However, each actor alone in the relationship has the power to transform the way in which the script of the medical visit is written. We have seen, in our review of the research done in this field, that interventions directed toward patients, but without provider involvement, have been effective in achieving significant changes in the way in which the visit is conducted. Likewise, programs designed to change physician behavior have led to dramatic differences in the communication of the visit. While rare, such interventions would be all the more successful if they were to simultaneously address both participants in the medical encounter.

The most successful patient interventions are those that foster and encourage a partnership on the part of patients and physicians—a partnership based on the patient's confidence in his or her own self-knowledge and ability to take an active and competent role in his or her own medical affairs. For physicians, we believe that the most effective interventions are also those that foster a partnership based on an acknowledgment of the unique store of experience and insight possessed by the patient, which can be as crucial for a positive treatment outcome as the physician's biomedical knowledge. There is a need for physicians to recognize that "apples are red and sweet as well as being composed of cells and molecules" (K. L. White, 1988, p. 6)—that a patient's experience of life is more than the function of his or her body systems.

The medical community is of two minds when considering issues of the doctor-patient relationship. The centrality of the doctor-patient relationship to patient care is among the oldest of themes in the history of medicine, dating back to the time of Hippocrates. Public concern for the quality of the therapeutic relationship is no less in modern times. Indeed, this concern has led to at least token acknowledgment of the relationship in the incorporation of courses dealing with this topic into the curriculum of most major medical schools. Yet, for many physicians, it is technology and the scientific method, divorced from issues of the therapeutic relationship, that are viewed as the *sine qua non* of medicine; in the real practice of medicine, many maintain, the issues of the doctor-patient relationship are relegated to an inconsequential and unscientific low-priority concern.

Just as in the first edition of this book, we end with optimism. We have been fortunate to work with an ever growing group of researchers and clinicians who are committed to the principles of relationship-centered care. While working on the fringes of medicine 20 years ago, our friends and colleagues are now part of the influential mainstream of American medicine. Many have taken leadership roles in studying and teaching about communication processes to medical students and other physicians throughout the world; as mentors and role models, such physician-teachers are shaping the attitudes and knowledge of the next professional generation. With relationships at its center, we believe that medical care will flourish. True respect will characterize the exchange, collaboration will replace medical authority, and the wisdom of both biomedical and social science will be applied to preserving that delicate balance we call health.

Bibliography

Aikin, K. J., Swasy, J. L., & Braman, A. C. (2004). Patient and physician attitudes and behaviors associated with DTC promotion of prescription drugs: Summary of FDA survey research results. Office of Medical Policy, Division of Drug Marketing, Advertising, and Communications. Washington, DC. Available at http://www.fda.gov/cder/ddmac/Final%20Report/FRFinalExSu119042. pdf (accessed February 5, 2006).

Ainsworth, M. A., Rogers, L. P., Markus, J. F., Dorsey, N. K., Blackwell, T. A., & Petrusa, E. R. (1991). Standardized patient encounters: A method for teaching and evaluation. *Journal of the American Medical Association, 266,* 1390–1396.

Albanese, M. A., Snow, M. H., Skochelak, S. E., Huggett, K. N., & Farrell, P. M. (2003). Assessing personal qualities in medical school admissions. *Academic Medicine, 78,* 313–321.

Ambady, N., LaPlante, D., Nguyen, T., Rosenthal, R., Chaumeton, N., & Levinson, W. (2002). Surgeons' tone of voice: A clue to malpractice history. *Surgery, 132,* 5–9.

Arora, N. K., & McHorney, C. A. (2000). Patient preferences for medical decision-making: Who really wants to participate? *Medical Care, 38,* 335–341.

Asch, D., & Parker, R. (1988). The Libby Zion case. *New England Journal of Medicine, 318,* 771–774.

Ashworth, C. K., Williamson, P., & Montano, D. (1984). A scale to measure physician beliefs about psychosocial aspects of patient care. *Social Science & Medicine, 19,* 1235–1238.

Bach, P. B., Pham, H. H., Schrag, D., Tate, R. C., & Hargraves, J. L. (2004). Primary care physicians who treat blacks and whites. *New England Journal of Medicine, 351*, 575–584.

Baile, W. F., Kudelka, A. P., Beale, E. A., Glober, G. A., Myers, E. G., Greisinger, A. J., et al. (1999). Communication skills training in oncology: Description and preliminary outcomes of workshops on breaking bad news and managing patient reactions to illness. *Cancer, 86*, 887–897.

Bain, D. J. (1979). The content of physician/patient communication in family practice. *Journal of Family Practice, 8*, 745–753.

Baker, D. W., Parker, R. M., Williams, M. V., Pitkin, K., Parikh, N. S., Coates, W., et al. (1996). The health care experience of patients with low literacy. *Archives of Family Medicine, 5*, 329–334.

Baker, D. W., Gazmararian, J. A., Sudano, J., Patterson, M., Parker, R. M., & Williams, M. V. (2002). Health literacy and performance on the Mini-Mental State Examination. *Aging and Mental Health, 6*, 22–29.

Baker, L., Wagner, T. H., Singer, S., & Bundorf, M. K. (2003). Use of the internet and e-mail for health care information: Results from a national survey. *Journal of the American Medical Association, 289*, 2400–2406.

Bales, R. F. (1950). *Interaction process analysis.* Cambridge, England: Addison-Wesley.

Barber, B. (1980). *Informed consent in medical therapy and research.* New Brunswick, NJ: Rutgers University Press.

Baron, R. M., & Kenny, D. A. (1986). The moderator-mediator variable distinction in social psychological research: Conceptual, strategic, and statistical considerations. *Journal of Personality and Social Psychology, 51*, 1173–1182.

Barrows, H. S. (1993). An overview of the uses of standardized patients for teaching and evaluating clinical skills. *Academic Medicine, 68*, 443–451.

Barsky, A. J. (1981). Hidden reasons some patients visit doctors. *Annals of Internal Medicine, 94*, 492–498.

Bartlett, E. E., Grayson, M., Barker, R., Levine, D. M., Golden, A., & Libber, S. (1984). The effects of physician communication skills on patient satisfaction, recall, and adherence. *Journal of Chronic Diseases, 37*, 755–764.

Barzansky, B., Jonas, H. S., & Etzel, S. I. (2000). Educational programs in U.S. medical schools, 1999–2000. *Journal of the American Medical Association, 284*, 1114–1120.

Barzini, L. (1965). *The Italians.* New York: Bantam Press.

Bass, M. J., Buck, C., Turner, L., Dickie, G., Pratt, G., & Robinson, H. C. (1986). The physician's actions and the outcome of illness in family practice. *Journal of Family Practice, 23*, 43–47.

Bass, P. F., III, Wilson, J. F., Griffith, C. H., & Barnett, D. R. (2002). Residents' ability to identify patients with poor literacy skills. *Academic Medicine, 77*, 1039–41.

Batenburg, V., Smal, J. A., Lodder, A., & de Melker, R. A. (1999). Are professional attitudes related to gender and medical specialty? *Medical Education, 33*, 489–492.

Baur, C. (2000). Limiting factors on the transformative powers of e-mail in patient-physician relationships: A critical analysis. *Health Communication, 12*, 239–259.

Baur, C. (2004). The Internet and health literacy: Moving beyond the brochure. In J. Schwartzberg, J. Van Geest, C. Wang, J. Gazmararian, R. Parker, D. Roter, R. Rudd, and D. Schillinger (Eds.). *Understanding health literacy: Implications for medicine and public health.* Chicago, IL: AMA Press.

Beach, M. C., & Inui, T., with the Relationship-Centered Care Research Network (2006). Relationship-centered care: A constructive reframing. *Journal of General Internal Medicine, 21* Suppl 1:S3–S8.

Beckman, H. B., & Frankel, R. M. (1984). The effect of physician behavior on the collection of data. *Annals of Internal Medicine, 101*, 692–696.

Beckman, H. B., Markakis, K. M., Suchman, A. L., & Frankel, R. M. (1994). The doctor-plaintiff relationship: Lessons from plaintiff depositions. *Archives of Internal Medicine, 154*, 1365–1370.

Beisecker, A. E. (1989). The influence of a companion on the doctor-elderly patient interaction. *Health Communication, 1*, 55–70.

Bensing, J. M., Kerssens, J. J., & van der Pasch, M. (1995). Patient-directed gaze as a tool for discovering and handling psychosocial problems in general practice. *Journal of Nonverbal Behavior, 19*, 223–242.

Bensing, J. M., Roter, D. L., & Hulsman, R. L. (2003). Communication patterns of primary care physicians in the U.S. and the Netherlands. *Journal of General Internal Medicine, 18*, 335–342.

Bensing, J. M., & Sluijs, E. M. (1985). Evaluation of an interview training course for general practitioners. *Social Science & Medicine, 20*, 737–744.

Bensing, J. M., van den Brink-Muinen, A., & de Bakker, D. H. (1993). Gender differences in practice style: A Dutch study of general practitioners. *Medical Care, 31*, 219–229.

Bernstein, B., & Kane, R. (1981). Physicians' attitudes toward female patients. *Medical Care, 19*, 600–608.

Bernzweig, J., Takayama, J. I., Phibbs, C., Lewis, C., & Pantell, R. H. (1997). Gender differences in physician-patient communication: Evidence from pediatric visits. *Archives of Pediatric and Adolescent Medicine, 151*, 586–591.

Bertakis, K. D., Callahan, E. J., Helms, L. J., Azari, R., Robbins, J. A., & Miller, J. (1998). Physician practice styles and patient outcomes: Differences between family practice and general internal medicine. *Medical Care, 36*, 879–891.

Bertakis, K. D., Helms, L. J., Callahan, E. J., Azari, R., & Robbins, J. A. (1995). The influence of gender on physician practice style. *Medical Care, 33*, 407–416.

Bertakis, K. D., Roter, D., & Putnam, S. M. (1991). The relationship of physician medical interview style to patient satisfaction. *Journal of Family Practice, 32*, 175–181.

Biener, L. (1983). Perceptions of patients by emergency room staff: Substance-abusers vs. non substance abusers. *Journal of Health and Social Behavior, 24*, 264–275.

Boon, H., & Stewart, M. (1998). Patient-physician communication assessment instruments: 1986 to 1996 in review. *Patient Education and Counseling, 35*, 161–176.

Boreham, P., & Gibson, D. (1978). The informative process in private medical consultations: A preliminary investigation. *Social Science & Medicine, 12*, 409–416.

Brody, D. S. (1980). The patient's role in clinical decision-making. *Annals of Internal Medicine, 93*, 718–722.

Bronson, D. L., Costanza, M. C., & Tufo, H. M. (1986). Using medical records for older patient education in ambulatory practice. *Medical Care, 24*, 332–339.

Brown, H. C., & Smith, H. J. (2004). Giving women their own case notes to carry during pregnancy. *The Cochrane Database of Systematic Reviews.* Issue 2. Art. No.: CD002856.pub2.DOI: 10.1002/14561858.PUB2.

Brown, J. B., Stewart, M. A., McCracken, E. C., McWhinney, I. R., & Levenstein, J. H. (1986). The patient-centered clinical method: 2. Definition and application. *Family Practice, 3*, 75–79.

Brown, J. B., Stewart, M., & Tessier, S. (1995). Assessing communication between patients and doctors: A manual for scoring patient-centered communication. Working paper series (Paper No. 95). University of Western Ontario, Centre for Studies in Family Medicine, London, Ontario, Canada.

Brown, J. B., Weston, W. W., & Stewart, M. A. (1989). Patient-centered interviewing. Part II: Finding common ground. *Canadian Family Physician, 35*, 153–157.

Buller, M. K., & Buller, D. B. (1985). Physicians' communication style and patient satisfaction. *Journal of Health and Social Behavior, 28*, 375–388.

Burgoon, J. K., Pfau, M., Parrott, R., Birk, T., Coker, R., & Burgoon, M. (1987). Relational communication, satisfaction, compliance-gaining strategies, and compliance in communication between physicians and patients. *Communication Monographs, 54*, 307–324.

Butterfield, P. (1988). The stress of residency: A review of the literature. *Archives of Internal Medicine, 148*, 1428–1435.

Byrne, J. M., & Long, B. E. L. (1976). *Doctors talking to patients.* London: Her Majesty's Stationery Office.

Caporael, L. R. (1981). The paralanguage of caregiving: Baby talk to the institutional-ized aged. *Journal of Personality and Social Psychology, 40*, 876–884.

Caporael, L. R., Lukaszewski, M. P., & Culbertson, G. H. (1983). Secondary baby talk: Judgments by institutionalized elderly and their caregivers. *Journal of Personality and Social Psychology, 44*, 746–756.

Carr, P. L, Gareis, K. C., & Barnett, R. C. (2003). Characteristics and outcomes for women physicians who work reduced hours. *Journal of Women's Health, 12,* 399–405.

Carrese, J. A., & Rhodes, L. A. (2000). Bridging cultural differences in medical practice: The case of discussing negative information with Navajo patients. *Journal of General Internal Medicine, 15,* 92–96.

Carr-Hill, R., Jenkins-Clarke, S., Dixon, P., & Pringle, M. (1998). Do minutes count? Consultation lengths in general practice. *Journal of Health Services Research and Policy, 3,* 207–213.

Cartwright, A. (1964). *Human relations and hospital care.* London: Routledge & Kegan Paul.

Cath, T., Graham, J., Potts, H. W. W., Richards, M. A., & Ramirez, A. J. (2005). Changes in mental health of UK hospital consultants since the mid-1990's. *Lancet, 366,* 742–744.

Cegala, D. J., McGee, D. S., & McNeilis, K. S. (1996). Components of patients' and doctors' perceptions of communication competence during a primary care medical interview. *Health Communication, 8,* 1–27.

Chen, F. M., Fryer, G. E., Philips, R. L., Wilson, E., & Pathman, D. E. (2005). Patients' beliefs about racism, preferences for physician race, and satisfaction with care. *Annals of Family Medicine, 3,* 138–143.

Christy, N. P. (1979). English is our second language. *New England Journal of Medicine, 300,* 979–981.

Clayman, M. L., Roter, D. L., Wissow, L. S., & Bandeen-Roche, K. (2005). Autonomy-related behaviors of patient companions and their effect on decision-making activity in geriatric primary care visits. *Social Science & Medicine, 60,* 1583–1591.

Coe, R. M. (1970). *Sociology of medicine.* New York: McGraw-Hill.

Cohen-Cole, S. (1991). *The medical interview: The three function approach.* St. Louis, MO: Mosby.

Cole-Kelly, K. (1994). Cultures engaging cultures: International medical graduates training in the United States. *Family Medicine, 26,* 618–624.

Coleman, T., & Manku-Scott, T. (1998). Comparison of video-recorded consultations with those in which patients' consent is withheld. *British Journal of General Practice, 48,* 971–974.

Collins, K. S., Hughes, D. L., Doty, M. M., Ives, B. L., Edwards, J. N., Tenney, K. (2002). *Diverse communities, common concerns: Assessing health care quality for minority Americans. Findings from The Commonwealth Fund 2001 Health Care Quality Survey.* New York: The Commonwealth Fund.

Cooper, L. A., & Roter, D. L. (2003). Patient-provider communication: The effect of race and ethnicity on process and outcomes of health care. In B. D. Smedley, A. Y. Stith, & A. R. Nelson (Eds.), *Unequal treatment: Confronting racial and ethnic disparities in health care* (pp. 552–593). Washington, DC: National Academies Press.

Cooper, L. A., Roter, D. L., Johnson. R. L., Ford, D. E., Steinwachs, D. M., & Powe, N. R. (2003). Patient-centered communication, ratings of care, and concordance of patient and physician race. *Annals of Internal Medicine, 139*, 907–915.

Cooper, R. A. (2003). Impact of trends in primary, secondary, and postsecondary education on applications to medical school II: Considerations of race, ethnicity, and income. *Academic Medicine, 78*, 864–876.

Cousins, N. (1979). *Anatomy of an illness as perceived by the patient.* New York: Norton.

Crandall, S. J., Volk, R. J., & Loemker, V. (1993). Medical students' attitudes toward providing care for the underserved: Are we training socially responsible physicians? *Journal of the American Medical Association, 19*, 2519–2523.

Cull, W. L., Mulvey, H. J., O'Connor, K. G., Sowell, D. R., Berkowitz, C. D., & Britton, C. V. (2002). Pediatricians working part-time: Past, present, future. *Pediatrics, 19*, 1015–1020.

Daugherty, S. R., Baldwin, D. C., & Rowley, B. D. (1998). Learning, satisfaction, and mistreatment during medical internship. *Journal of the American Medical Association, 279*, 1194–1199.

Davis, T., Crouch, M., Wills, G., Miller, S., & Adebhou, D. (1990). The gap between patient reading comprehension and the readability of patient education materials. *Journal of Family Practice, 31*, 533–538.

Delbanco, T., & Sands, D. Z. (2004). Electrons in flight—E-mail between doctors and patients. *New England Journal of Medicine, 350*, 1705–1707.

de Ridder, D., Fournier, M., & Bensing, J. (2004). Does optimism affect symptom report in chronic disease? What are its consequences for self-care behavior and physical functioning? *Journal of Psychosomatic Research, 56*, 341–350.

Devine, E. C. (1992). Effects of psychoeducational care for adult surgical patients: A meta-analysis of 191 studies. *Patient Education and Counseling, 19*, 129–142.

DiMatteo, M. R. (1994). Enhancing patient adherence to medical recommendations. *Journal of the American Medical Association, 271*, 79–83.

DiMatteo, M. R. (2004). Variations in patients' adherence to medical recommendations: A quantitative review of 50 years of research. *Medical Care, 42*, 200–209.

DiMatteo, M. R., & DiNicola, D. D. (1982). *Achieving patient compliance.* New York: Pergamon Press.

DiMatteo, M. R., Giordani, P. J., Lepper, H. S., & Croghan, T. W. (2002). Patient adherence and medical treatment outcomes: A meta-analysis. *Medical Care, 40*, 794–811.

DiMatteo, M. R., Hays, R. D., & Prince, L. M. (1986). Relationship of physicians' nonverbal communication skill to patient satisfaction, appointment non-compliance, and physician workload. *Health Psychology, 5*, 581–594.

DiMatteo, M. R., Reiter, R. C., & Gambone, J. C. (1994). Enhancing medication adherence through communication and informed collaborative choice. *Health Communication, 6*, 253–265.

DiMatteo, M. R., Taranta, A., Friedman, H. S., & Prince, L. M. (1980). Predicting patient satisfaction from physicians' nonverbal communication skills. *Medical Care, 18*, 376–387.

Dindia, K., & Allen, M. (1992). Sex differences in self-disclosure: A meta-analysis. *Psychological Bulletin, 112*, 106–124.

Dorsey, E. R., Jarjoura, D., & Rutecki, G. W. (2005). The influence of controllable lifestyle and sex on the specialty choices of graduating U.S. medical students, 1996–2003. *Academic Medicine, 80*, 791–796.

Drew, J., Stoeckle, J. D., & Billings, J. A. (1983). Tips, status and sacrifice: Gift giving in the doctor-patient relationship. *Social Science & Medicine, 17*, 399–404.

Dungal, L. (1978). Physicians' responses to patients: A study of factors involved in the office interview. *Journal of Family Practice, 6*, 1065–1073.

Eagly, A. H., & Johnson, B. T. (1990). Gender and leadership style: A meta-analysis. *Psychological Bulletin, 108*, 233–256.

Educational Commission for Foreign Medical Graduates (2002). *Annual report: Committed to promoting excellence in international medical education.* http://www.ecfmg.org/annuals/2002/index.html

Egbert, L. D., Battit, G. E., Welch, C. E., & Bartlett, M. K. (1964). Reduction of postoperative pain by encouragement and instruction of patients. *New England Journal of Medicine, 270*, 825–827.

Eisenberg, J. M. (1979). Sociologic influences on decision making by clinicians. *Annals of Internal Medicine, 90*, 957–964.

Eisenberg, J. (1986). *Doctors' decisions and the cost of medical care.* Ann Arbor: Health Administration Press.

Elstad, J. I. (1994). Women's priorities regarding physician behavior and their preference for a female physician. *Women & Health, 21*, 1–19.

Emanuel, E. J., & Emanuel, L. L. (1992). Four models of the physician-patient relationship. *Journal of the American Medical Association, 267*, 2221–2226.

Ende, J., Kazis, L., Ash, A., & Moskowitz, M. A. (1989). Measuring patients' desire for autonomy: Decision making and information-seeking preferences among medical patients. *Journal of General Internal Medicine, 4*, 23–30.

Ende, J., Kazis, L., & Moskowitz, M. A. (1990). Preferences for autonomy when patients are physicians. *Journal of General Internal Medicine, 5*, 506–509.

Engel, G. L. (1977). The need for a new medical model: A challenge for biomedicine. *Science, 196*, 129–136.

Epstein, A. M., Begg, C. B., & McNeil, B. J. (1984). The effects of physicians' training and personality on test ordering for ambulatory patients. *American Journal of Public Health, 74*, 1271–1273.

Epstein, A. M., Hall, J. A., Tognetti, J., Son, L. H., & Conant, L., Jr. (1989). Using proxies to evaluate quality of life: Can they provide valid information about patients' health status and satisfaction with medical care? *Medical Care, 27*, S91–S98.

Epstein, A. M., Taylor, W. C., & Seage, G .R. (1985). Effects of patients' socioeconomic status and physicians' training and practice on patient-doctor communication. *American Journal of Medicine, 78*, 101–106.

Evans, B. J., Kiellerup, F. D., Stanley, R. O., Burrows, G. D., & Sweet, B. (1987). A communication skills programme for increasing patients' satisfaction with general practice consultations. *British Journal of Medical Psychology, 60*, 373–378.

Faden, R., Becker, C., Lewis, C., Freeman, J., & Faden, A. (1981). Disclosure of information to patients in medical care. *Medical Care, 19*, 718–733.

Fallowfield, L. J. (1995). Can we improve the professional and personal fulfillment of doctors in cancer medicine? *British Journal of Cancer, 71*, 1132–1133.

Fallowfield, L. J., Baum, M., & Maguire, G. P. (1986). Effects of breast conservation on psychological morbidity associated with diagnosis and treatment of early breast cancer. *British Medical Journal, 293*, 1331–1334.

Fallowfield, L. J., Hall, A., Maguire, G. P., & Baum, M. (1990). Psychological outcomes of different treatment policies in women with early breast cancer outside a clinical trial. *British Medical Journal, 301*, 575–580.

Fallowfield, L. J., & Jenkins, V. (1999). Effective communication skills are the key to good cancer care. *European Journal of Cancer, 35*, 1592–1597.

Ferguson, T. (1998). Digital doctoring-opportunities and challenges in electronic patient-physician communication. *Journal of the American Medical Association, 280*, 1361–1362.

Festinger, L. (1957). *A theory of cognitive dissonance.* Stanford, CA: University of California Press.

Fine, V. K., & Therrien, M. E. (1977). Empathy in the doctor-patient relationship: Skill training for medical students. *Journal of Medical Education, 52*, 152–157.

Fiscella, K., Roman-Diaz, M., Bee-Horng, L., Botelho, R., & Frankel, R. (1997). "Being a foreigner, I may be punished if I make a small mistake": Assessing transcultural experiences in caring for patients. *Family Practice, 14*, 112–116.

Fischback, R. L., Bayog, A. S., Needle, A., & Delbanco, T. L. (1980). The patient and practitioner as co-authors of the medical record. *Patient Counseling and Health Education, 2*, 1–5.

Fogarty, L. A., Curbow, B. A., Wingard, J. R., McDonnell, K., & Somerfield, M. R. (1999). Can 40 seconds of compassion reduce patient anxiety? *Journal of Psychosocial Oncology, 17*, 371–379.

Fortinsky, R. H. (2001). Health care triads and dementia care: Integrative framework and future directions. *Aging and Mental Health, 5*(Suppl 1), S35–S48.

Fox, J. G., & Storms, D. M. (1981). A different approach to sociodemographic predictors of satisfaction with health care. *Social Science & Medicine, 15A*, 557–564.

Fox, R. (1989). *Essays in medical sociology: Journeys into the field.* New Brunswick, NJ: Transaction Books.

Fox, S. (2003). Opportunities and challenges: Using the Internet for prevention. *Pew Internet and the American Life Project* (http://www.pewinternet.org).

Fox, S., & Fallows, D. (2003). Internet Health Resources. *Pew Internet & American Life Project* (http://www.pewinternet.org).

Frederikson, L. G. (1993). Development of an integrative model for medical consultation. *Health Communication, 5*, 225–237.

Freeman, S. H. (1987). Health promotion talk in family practice encounters. *Social Science & Medicine, 25*, 961–966.

Freemon, B., Negrete, V., Davis, M., & Korsch, B. (1971). Gaps in doctor patient communication. *Pediatric Research, 5*, 298–311.

Freidson, E. (1960). Client control and medical practice. *American Journal of Sociology, 65*, 374–382.

Freidson, E. (1970). *Professional dominance.* Chicago: Aldine Press.

Freidson, E. (1975). *Doctoring together: A study of professional social control.* New York: Elsevier.

Freire, P. (1970). *Pedagogy of the oppressed.* New York: Seabury Press.

Friedman, H. S., Hall, J. A., & Harris, M. J. (1985). Type A behavior, nonverbal expressive style, and health. *Journal of Personality and Social Psychology, 48*, 1299–1315.

Fuller, S., Endress, P. L., & Johnson, J. (1978). The effects of cognitive and behavioral control on coping with an aversive health examination. *Journal of Human Stress,* December, 18–25.

Gladwin, T. (1964). Culture and logical process. In W. H. Goodenough (Ed.), *Explorations in cultural anthropology: Essays in honor of George Peter Mudock* (pp. 167–177). New York: McGraw Hill.

Goldstein, S., Fischer, P. M., Richards, J. W., Goldstein, A., & Shank, J. C. (1987). Smoking counseling practices of recently trained family physicians. *Journal of Family Practice, 24*, 195–197.

Golin, C. E., DiMatteo, M. R., & Gelberg, L. (1996). The role of patient participation in the doctor visit: Implications for adherence to diabetes care. *Diabetes Care, 19*, 1153–1164.

Gotler, R. S., Flocke, S. A., Goodwin, M. A., Zyzanski, S. J., Murray, T. H., & Stange, K. C. (2000). Facilitating participatory decision-making: What happens in real-world community practice? *Medical Care, 38*, 1200–1209.

Greene, M. G., Adelman, R. D., Charon, R., & Friedmann, E. (1989). Concordance between physicians and their older and younger patients in the primary care medical encounter. *The Gerontologist, 29*, 808–813.

Greene, M. G., Adelman, R. D., Charon, R., & Hoffman, S. (1986). Ageism in the medical encounter: An exploratory study of the language and behavior of doctors with their old and young patients. *Language and Communication, 6*, 113–124.

Greene, M. G., Majerovitz, S. D., Adelman, R. D., & Rizzo, C. (1994). The effects of the presence of a third person on the physician-older patient medical interview. *Journal of the American Geriatric Society, 42*, 413–419.

Greenfield, S., Kaplan, S. H., & Ware, J. E., Jr. (1985). Expanding patient involvement in care: Effects on patient outcomes. *Annals of Internal Medicine, 102*, 520–528.

Greenfield, S., Kaplan, S. H., Ware, J. E. Jr., Yano, E. M., & Frank, H. J. (1988). Patients' participation in medical care: Effects on blood sugar control and quality of life in diabetes. *Journal of General Internal Medicine, 3*, 448–457.

Griffin, S. J., Kinmonth, A-L., Veltman, M. W. M., Gillard, S., Grant, J., & Stewart, M. (2004). Effect on health-related outcomes of interventions to alter the interaction between patients and practitioners: A systematic review of trials. *Annals of Family Medicine, 2*, 595–608.

Griffith, C. H., Haist, S. A., Wilson, J. F., & Rich, E. C. (1996). Housestaff social history knowledge: Correlation with evaluation of interpersonal skills. *Evaluation and the Health Professions, 19*, 81–90.

Griffith, C. H., Rich, E. C., & Wilson, J. F. (1995). Housestaff knowledge of their patient's social history. *Academic Medicine, 70*, 64–69.

Griffith, C. H. III, Wilson, J. F. (2001). The loss of student idealism in the third year clinical clerkships. *Evaluation and the Health Professions, 24*, 61–71.

Groves, J. E. (1978). Taking care of the hateful patient. *New England Journal of Medicine, 298*, 883–887.

Haezen-Klemens, I., & Lapinska, E. (1984). Doctor-patient interaction, patients' health behaviour and effects of treatment. *Social Science & Medicine, 19*, 9–18.

Hafferty, F. W. (1998). Beyond curriculum reform: Confronting medicine's hidden curriculum. *Academic Medicine, 73*, 403–407.

Hagedoorn, M., Uijl, S. G., Van Sonderen, E., Ranchor, A. V., Grol, B. M. F., Otter, R., et al. (2003). Structure and reliability of Ware's Patient Satisfaction Questionnaire III: Patients' satisfaction with oncological care in the Netherlands. *Medical Care, 41*, 254–263.

Haidet, P., Dains, J. E., Paterniti, D. A., Hechtel, L., Chang, T., Tseng, E., & Rogers, J. C. (2002). Medical student attitudes toward the doctor-patient relationship. *Medical Education, 46*, 568–574.

Hall, E. T. *Beyond culture.* (1976). Garden City, NY: Anchor Press/Doubleday.

Hall, J. A. (1984). *Nonverbal sex differences: Communication accuracy and expressive style.* Baltimore: Johns Hopkins University Press.

Hall, J. A. (2006). Women's and men's nonverbal communication: Similarities, differences, stereotypes, and origins. In V. Manusov & M. L. Patterson (Eds.), *The SAGE handbook of nonverbal communication*. Thousand Oaks, CA: Sage, 201–218.

Hall, J. A., & Braunwald, K. G. (1981). Gender cues in conversations. *Journal of Personality and Social Psychology, 40*, 99–110.

Hall, J. A., & Dornan, M. C. (1988a). Meta-analysis of satisfaction with medical care: Description of research domains and analysis of overall satisfaction levels. *Social Science & Medicine, 27*, 637–644.

Hall, J. A., & Dornan, M. C. (1988b). What patients like about their medical care and how often they are asked: A meta-analysis of the satisfaction literature. *Social Science & Medicine, 27*, 935–939.

Hall, J. A., & Dornan, M. C. (1990). Patient sociodemographic characteristics as predictors of satisfaction with medical care: A meta-analysis. *Social Science & Medicine, 30*, 811–818.

Hall, J. A., Epstein, A. M., DeCiantis, M., & McNeil, B. J. (1993). Physicians' liking for their patients: Further evidence for the role of affect in medical care. *Health Psychology, 12*, 140–146.

Hall, J. A., Epstein, A. M., & McNeil, B. J. (1989). Multidimensionality of health status in an elderly population: Construct validity of a measurement battery. *Medical Care, 27*, S168–S177.

Hall, J. A., Feldstein, M., Fretwell, M. D., Rowe, J. W., & Epstein, A. M. (1990). Older patients' health status and satisfaction with medical care in an HMO population. *Medical Care, 28*, 261–270.

Hall, J. A., Friedman, H. S., & Harris, M. J. (1986). Nonverbal cues, the Type A behavior pattern, and coronary heart disease. In P. D. Blanck, R. Buck, & R. Rosenthal (Eds.), *Nonverbal communication in the clinical context* (pp. 144–168). State College, PA: Pennsylvania State University Press.

Hall, J. A., Harrigan, J. A., & Rosenthal, R. (1995). Nonverbal behavior in clinician-patient interaction. *Applied and Preventive Psychology, 4*, 21–37.

Hall, J. A., Horgan, T. G., Stein, T. S., & Roter, D. L. (2002). Liking in the physician-patient relationship. *Patient Education and Counseling, 48*, 69–77.

Hall, J. A., Irish, J. T., Roter, D. L., Ehrlich, C. M., & Miller, L. H. (1994a). Gender in medical encounters: An analysis of physician and patient communication in a primary care setting. *Health Psychology, 13*, 384–392.

Hall, J. A., Irish, J. T., Roter, D. L., Ehrlich, C. M., & Miller, L. H. (1994b). Satisfaction, gender, and communication in medical visits. *Medical Care, 32*, 1216–1231.

Hall, J. A., Milburn, M. A., Roter, D. L., & Daltroy, L. H. (1998). Why are sicker patients less satisfied with their care? Tests of two explanatory models. *Health Psychology, 17*, 70–75.

Hall, J. A., Palmer, R. H., Orav, E. J., Hargraves, J. L., Wright, E. A., & Louis, T. A. (1990). Performance quality, gender, and professional role: A study of physicians and nonphysicians in 16 ambulatory care practices. *Medical Care, 28*, 489–501.

Hall, J. A., & Roter, D. L. (1995). Patient gender and communication with physicians: Results of a community-based study. *Women's Health: Research on Gender, Behavior, and Policy, 1*, 77–95.

Hall, J. A., & Roter, D. L. (2002). Do patients talk differently to male and female physicians? A meta-analytic review. *Patient Education and Counseling, 48*, 217–224.

Hall, J. A., Roter, D. L., & Katz, N. R. (1987). Task versus socioemotional behaviors in physicians. *Medical Care, 25*, 399–412.

Hall, J. A., Roter, D. L., & Katz, N. R. (1988). Meta-analysis of correlates of provider behavior in medical encounters. *Medical Care, 26*, 657–675.

Hall, J. A., Roter, D. L., Milburn, M. A., & Daltroy, L. H. (1996). Patients' health as a predictor of physician and patient behavior in medical visits: A synthesis of four studies. *Medical Care, 34*, 1205–1218.

Hall, J. A., Roter, D. L., & Rand, C. S. (1981). Communication of affect between patient and physician. *Journal of Health and Social Behavior, 22*, 18–30.

Hall, J. A., & Schmid Mast, M. (2004). Five ways of being theoretical: Applications to provider-patient communication research. Unpublished manuscript, Northeastern University, Boston, MA.

Hall, J. A., Stein, T. S., Roter, D. L., & Rieser, N. (1999). Inaccuracies in physicians' perceptions of their patients. *Medical Care, 37*, 1164–1168.

Handler, A., Rosenberg, D., Raube, K., & Kelley, M. A. (1998). Health care characteristics associated with women's satisfaction with prenatal care. *Medical Care, 36*, 679–694.

Harden, J. (2001). "Mother Russia" at work: Gender division in the medical profession. *European Journal of Women's Studies, 8*, 181–199.

Harrington, J., Noble, L. M., & Newman, S. P. (2004). Improving patients' communication with doctors: A systematic review of intervention studies. *Patient Education and Counseling, 52*, 7–16.

Harris Interactive (http://www.harrisinteractive.com/news/newsletters_healthcare.asp).

Hasselkus, B. R. (1988). Meaning in family caregiving: Perspectives on caregiver/professional relationships. *Gerontologist, 28*, 686–691.

Haug, M. R. (Ed.) (1981). *Elderly patients and their doctors.* New York: Springer Publishing Company.

Haug, M. R., & Lavin, B. (1981). Practitioner or patient—Who's in charge? *Journal of Health and Social Behavior, 22*, 212–229.

Haug, M., & Lavin, B. (1983). *Consumerism in medicine: Challenging physician authority.* Beverly Hills: Sage Publications.

Headache Study Group of the University of Western Ontario. (1986). Predictors of outcome in headache patients presenting to family physicians—a one year prospective study. *Headache, 26,* 285–294.

Heath, C. (1986). *Body movement and speech in medical interaction.* Cambridge, UK: Cambridge University Press.

Heath, C. (2002). Demonstrative suffering: The gestural (re)embodiment of symptoms. *Journal of Communication, 52,* 597–616.

Hedges, L. V., & Cooper, H. (Eds.). (1993). *Handbook of research synthesis.* New York: Russell Sage.

Heiligers, P. J. M., & Hingstman, L. (2000). Career preferences and the work-family balance in medicine: Gender differences among medical specialists. *Social Science & Medicine, 50,* 1235–1246.

Helfer, R. E. (1970). An objective comparison of the pediatric interviewing skills of freshman and senior medical students. *Pediatrics, 45,* 623–627.

Helft, P. R., Hlubocky, F., & Daugherty, C. K. (2003). American oncologists' views of internet use by cancer patients: A mail survey of American Society of Clinical Oncology members. *Journal of Clinical Oncology, 21,* 942–947.

Henbest, R. J., & Stewart, M. A. (1989). Patient-centeredness in the consultation I: A method for measurement. *Family Practice, 6,* 249–253.

Henderson, J. T., & Weisman, C. S. (2001). Physician gender effects on preventive screening and counseling: An analysis of male and female patients' health care experiences. *Medical Care, 39,* 1281–1292.

Hibbard, J. H., & Weeks, E. C. (1985). Consumer use of physician fee information. *Journal of Health and Human Resources Administration, 7,* 321–335.

Hibbard, J. H., & Weeks, E. C. (1987). Consumerism in health care: Prevalence and predictors. *Medical Care, 25,* 1019–1032.

Hickson, G. B., Clayton, E. W., & Entman, S. S. (1994). Obstetricians' prior malpractice experience and patients' satisfaction with care. *Journal of the American Medical Association, 272,* 1583–1587.

Hickson, G. B., Clayton , E. W., Githens, P. B., & Sloan, F. A. (1992). Factors that prompted families to file medical malpractice claims following perinatal injuries. *Journal of the American Medical Association, 267,* 1359–1363.

Hickson, G. B., Federspiel, C. F., Pichert, J. W., Miller, C. S., Gauld-Jaeger, J., & Bost, P. (2002). Patient complaints and malpractice risk. *Journal of the American Medical Association, 287,* 2951–2957.

Hilfiker, D. (1985). *Healing the wounds: A physician looks at his work.* New York: Pantheon.

Hogbin, B., & Fallowfield, L. (1989). Getting it taped: The "bad news" consultation with cancer patients. *British Journal of Hospital Medicine, 41,* 330–333.

Holder, A. R. (1970). Informed consent: Its evolution. *Journal of the American Medical Association, 214,* 1181–1182.

Homer, C. S., Davis, G. K., & Everitt L. S. (1999). The introduction of a woman-held record into a hospital antenatal clinic: The bring your own records study. *Australian and New Zealand Journal of Obstetrics and Gynaecology, 39*, 54–57.

Hooper, E. M., Comstock, L. M., Goodwin, J. M., & Goodwin, J. S. (1982). Patient characteristics that influence physician behavior. *Medical Care, 20*, 630–638.

Howie, J. G., Heaney, D. J., & Maxwell, M. (1997). Measuring quality in general practice: Pilot study of a needs, process and outcome measure. *Occasional Papers, Royal College of General Practitioners.* i–xii, 1–32.

Hughs, D. (1982). Control in medical consultation: The organizing talk in a situation where co-participants have differential competence. *Sociology, 16*, 359–376.

Hull, F. M., & Hull, F. S. (1984). Time and the general practitioner: The patient's view. *Journal of the Royal College of General Practice, 34*, 71–75.

Idler, E. L., & Kasl, S. V. (1991). Health perceptions and survival: Do global evaluations of health status really predict mortality? *Journal of Gerontology, 46*, S55–S65.

Institute of Medicine (1999). *To err is human: Building a safer health system.* L. T. Kohn, J. M. Corrigan, & M. S. Donaldson (Eds.). Washington, DC: National Academies Press.

Institute of Medicine (2001). *Crossing the quality chasm: A new health system.* Washington, DC: National Academies Press.

Institute of Medicine (2003). *Unequal treatment: Confronting racial and ethnic disparities in health care.* Washington, DC: National Academies Press.

Inui, T. S., Carter, W. B., Kukull, W. A., & Haigh, V. H. (1982). Outcome-based doctor-patient interaction analysis: I. Comparison of techniques. *Medical Care, 10*, 535–549.

Inui, T. S., Yourtee, E. L., & Williamson, J. W. (1976). Improved outcomes in hypertension after physician tutorials: A controlled trial. *Annals of Internal Medicine, 84*, 646–651.

Jackson, J. L., Chamberlin, J., Kroenke, K. (2001). Predictors of patient satisfaction. *Social Science & Medicine, 52*, 609-620.

Jagsi, R., Shapiro, J., & Weinstein, D. F. (2005). Perceived impact of resident work hour limitations on medical student clerkships: A survey study. *Academic Medicine, 80*, 752–757.

Johnson, J., Kirchoff, K., & Endress, P. (1975). Altering children's distress behavior during orthopedic cast removal. *Nursing Research, 24*, 404–410.

Johnson, J., & Leventhal, H. (1974). Effects of accurate expectations and behavioral instructions on reactions during a noxious medical examination. *Journal of Personality and Social Psychology, 29*, 710–718.

Johnson, J. E., Nail, L. M., Lauver, D., King, K. B., & Keys, H. (1988). Reducing the negative impact of radiation therapy on functional status. *Cancer, 61*, 46–51.

Jolly, P. (2004). *Medical school tuition and young physician indebtedness.* Washington, DC: Association of American Medical Colleges.

Jonas, H. S., & Etzel, S. (1988). Undergraduate medical education. *Journal of the American Medical Association, 260,* 1063–1071.

Kain, Z. N., & Caldwell-Andrews, A. A. (2005). Preoperative psychological preparation of the child for surgery: An update. *Anesthesiology Clinics of North America, 23,* 597–614.

Kalisch, B. J. (1971). An experiment in the development of empathy in nursing students. *Nursing Research, 20,* 202–210.

Kaplan, S. H., Gandek, B., Greenfield, S., Rogers, W., & Ware, J. E. (1995). Patient and visit characteristics related to physicians' participatory decision-making style: Results from the Medical Outcomes Study. *Medical Care, 33,* 1176–1183.

Kaplan, S. H., Greenfield, S., Gandek, B., Rogers, W., & Ware, J. E. (1996). Characteristics of physicians with participatory decision-making styles. *Annals of Internal Medicine, 124,* 497–504.

Kaplan, S. H., Greenfield, S., & Ware, J. E. Jr. (1989). Assessing the effects of physician-patient interactions on the outcomes of chronic disease. *Medical Care, 27,* S110–S127.

Kiesler, D. J., & Auerbach, S. M. (2003). Integrating measurement of control and affiliation in studies of physician-patient interaction: The interpersonal circumplex. *Social Science & Medicine, 57,* 1707–1722.

Klass, P. (1987). *A not entirely benign procedure: Four years as a medical student.* New York: Signet.

Kleinman, A. (1987). Explanatory models in health care relationships: A conceptual frame for research on family-based health-care activities in relation to folk and professional forms of clinical care. In J. Stoeckle (Ed.), *Encounters between patients and doctors.* Cambridge, MA: MIT Press.

Knapp, M. L., & Hall, J. A. (2005). *Nonverbal communication in human interaction,* 6th ed. Belmont, CA: Wadsworth.

Koopman, C. S., Eisenthal, S., & Stoeckle, J. (1984). Ethnicity in the reported pain, emotional distress and requests of medical outpatients. *Social Science & Medicine, 6,* 487–490.

Koos, E. L. (1954). *The health of Regionville.* New York: Columbia University Press.

Korsch, B. M., Gozzi, E. K., & Francis, V. (1968). Gaps in doctor-patient communication: I. Doctor-patient interaction and patient satisfaction. *Pediatrics, 42,* 855–871.

Kramer, D., Ber, R., & Moore, M. (1987). Impact of workshop on students' and physicians' rejecting behaviors in patient interviews. *Journal of Medical Education, 62,* 904–910.

Kravitz, R. L. (2000). Direct-to-consumer advertising of prescription drugs. *Western Journal of Medicine, 173,* 221–222.

Kreps, G. L. (2001). Consumer/provider communication research: A personal plea to address issues of ecological validity, relational development, message diversity, and situational constraints. *Journal of Health Psychology, 6,* 597–601.

Krupat, E., Fancey, M., & Cleary, P. D. (2000). Information and its impact on satisfaction among surgical patients. *Social Science & Medicine, 51,* 1817–1825.

Krupat, E., Hiam, C. M., Fleming, M. Z., & Freeman, P. (1999). Patient-centeredness and its correlates among first year medical students. *International Journal of Psychiatry in Medicine, 29,* 347–356.

Krupat, E., Rosenkranz, S. L., Yeager, C. M., Barnard, K., Putnam, S. M., & Inui, T. S. (2000). The practice orientations of physicians and patients: The effect of doctor-patient congruence on satisfaction. *Patient Education and Counseling, 39,* 49–59.

Kubler-Ross, E. (1969). *On death and dying.* New York: McMillan Publishing Co.

Kulik, J. A., & Mahler, H. T. M. (1987). Effects of preoperative roommate assignment on preoperative anxiety and recovery from coronary-bypass surgery. *Health Psychology, 6,* 525–543.

Kulik, J. A., Mahler, H. I., & Moore, P. J. (1996). Social comparison and affiliation under threat: Effects on recovery from major surgery. *Journal of Personality and Social Psychology, 71,* 967–979.

Kulik, J. A., Moore, P. J., & Mahler, H. I. (1993). Stress and affiliation: Hospital roommate effects on preoperative anxiety and social interaction. *Health Psychology, 12,* 118–124.

Kurtz, R.A., & Chalfant, H. P. (1991). *The sociology of medicine and illness,* 2nd ed. Boston: Allyn & Bacon.

Kutner, B. (1972). Surgeons and their patients: A study in social perception. In E. G. Jaco (Ed.), *Patients, physicians and illness.* New York: Free Press.

Labrecque, M. S., Blanchard, C. G., Ruckdeschel, J. C., & Blanchard, E. B. (1991). The impact of family presence on the physician-cancer patient interaction. *Social Science & Medicine, 33,* 1253–1261.

Lamont, E. B., & Christakis, N. A. (2001). Prognostic disclosure to patients with cancer near the end of life. *Annals of Internal Medicine, 134,* 1096–1105.

Langer, E. J., & Rodin, J. (1976). The effects of choice and enhanced personal responsibility for the aged: A field experiment in an institutional setting. *Journal of Personality and Social Psychology, 34,* 191–198.

Larsson, U. S., Saljo, R., & Aronsson, K. (1987). Patient-doctor communication on smoking and drinking: Lifestyle in medical consultations. *Social Science & Medicine, 25,* 1129–1137.

Lasagna, L., Mosteller, F., von Feisinger, J. M., & Beecher, H. K. (1954). A study of the placebo response. *American Journal of Medicine, 37,* 770–779.

Laufenburg, H. F., Turkal, N. W., & Baumgardner, D. J. (1994). Resident attrition from family practice residencies: United States versus international medical graduates. *Family Medicine, 26*, 614–617.

Lazare, A. (1987). Shame and humiliation in the medical encounter. *Archives of Internal Medicine,147*, 1653–1658.

Lazare, A., Eisenthal, S., & Wasserman, L. (1975). The customer approach to patienthood: Attending to patient requests in a walk-in clinic. *Archives of General Psychiatry, 32*, 553–558.

Lazare, A., Putnam, S. M., & Lipkin, M., Jr. (1995). Three functions of the medical interview. In M. Lipkin, S. M. Putnam, & A. Lazare (Eds.), *The medical interview: Clinical care, education, and research* (pp. 3–19). New York: Springer-Verlag.

Lehmann, L. L., Brancati, F. L., Chen, M. C., Roter, D. L., & Dobs, A. S. (1997). The effect of bedside case presentations on patients' perceptions of their medical care. *New England Journal of Medicine, 336*, 1150–1155.

Leiderman, D. B., & Grisso, J. (1985). The GOMER phenomenon. *Journal of Health and Social Behavior, 26*, 222–232.

Leigh, J. P., Kravitz, R. L., Schembri, M., Samuels, S. J., & Mobley, S. (2002). Physician career satisfaction across specialties. *Archives of Internal Medicine, 162*, 1577–1584.

Levinson, W. (1993). Mining for gold. *Journal of General Internal Medicine, 8*, 172–174.

Levinson, W., & Lurie, N. (2004). When most doctors are women: what lies ahead? *Annals of Internal Medicine, 141*, 471–474.

Levinson, W., & Roter, D. L. (1995). Physicians' attitudes: The effect of communication with patients. *Journal of General Internal Medicine, 10*, 375–379.

Levinson, W., Roter, D. L., Mullooly, J., Dull, V., & Frankel, R. (1997). Doctor-patient communication: A critical link to malpractice in surgeons and primary care physicians. *Journal of the American Medical Association, 277*, 553–559.

Lewin, T. (2001). Women's health is no longer a man's world. *New York Times*, February 7, National Desk section.

Lewis, C. E., Lewis, M. A., Lorimer, A., & Palmer, B. B. (1977). Child-initiated care: The use of school nursing services by children in an "adult-free" system. *Pediatrics, 60*, 499–507.

Lewis, C. C., Scott, D. E., Pantell, R. H., & Wolf, M. H. (1986). Parent satisfaction with children's medical care: Development, field test, and validation of a questionnaire. *Medical Care, 24*, 209–215.

Light, D. (1975). The sociological calendar: An analytic tool for fieldwork applied to medical and psychiatric training. *American Journal of Sociology, 80*, 1145–1164.

Like, R., & Zyzanski, S. J. (1987). Patient satisfaction and the clinical encounter: Social psychological determinants. *Social Science & Medicine, 24*, 351–357.

Lindau, S. T., Tomori, C., McCarville, M. A., & Bennett, C. L. (2001). Improving rates of cervical cancer screening and Pap smear follow-up for low-income women with limited health literacy. *Cancer Investigation, 19*, 316–323.

Linn, B. S. (1982). Burn patients' evaluation of emergency department care. *Annals of Emergency Medicine, 11*, 255–259.

Linn, L. S., & Lewis, C. E. (1979). Attitudes toward self-care among practicing physicians. *Medical Care, 17*, 183–190.

Lipkin, M., Jr., Putnam, S. M., & Lazare, A. (Eds.) (1995). *The medical interview: Clinical care, education, and research.* New York: Springer-Verlag.

Lipkin, M., Jr., Putnam, S. M., & Lazare, A. (1995). Preface. In M. Lipkin, Jr., S. M. Putnam, & A. Lazare (Eds.), *The medical interview: Clinical care, education, and research* (pp. ix–xi). New York: Springer-Verlag.

Localio, A. R., Lawthers, A. G., & Brennan, T. A. (1991). Relation between malpractice claims and adverse events due to negligence: Results of the Harvard Medical Practice Study III. *New England Journal of Medicine, 325*, 245–251.

Lurie, N., Margolis, K. L., McGovern, P. G., Mink, P. J., & Slater, J. S. (1997). Why do patients of female physicians have higher rates of breast and cervical cancer screening? *Journal of General Internal Medicine, 12*, 34–43.

Maguire, P., Fairbairn, S., & Fletcher, C. (1989). Consultation skills of young doctors—benefits of undergraduate feedback training interviewing. In M. Stewart & D. Roter (Eds.), *Communicating with medical patients* (pp. 124–137). London: Sage.

Mahaffy, P. R. (1965). The effects of hospitalization on children admitted for tonsillectomy and adenoidectomy. *Nursing Research, 14*, 12–19.

Maheux, B., Dufort, F., Beland, F., Jacques, A., & Levesque, A. (1990). Female medical practitioners: More preventive and patient oriented? *Medical Care, 28*, 87–92.

Maheux, B., Pineault, R., & Beland, F. (1987). Factors influencing physicians' orientation toward prevention. *American Journal of Preventive Medicine, 3*, 12–18.

Maiman, L. A., Becker, M. H., Liptak, G. S., Nazarian, L. F., & Rounds, K. A. (1988). Improving pediatricians' compliance-enhancing practices: A randomized trial. *American Journal of Diseases of Children, 142*, 773–779.

Malat, J. (2001). Social distance and patients' rating of healthcare providers. *Journal of Health and Social Behavior, 42*, 360–372.

Manhattan Research, LLC. (2004). *Taking the pulse 4.0.* New York: Manhattan Research, LLC.

Marshal, V. W. (1981). Physician characteristics and relationships with older patients. In Haug, M. R. (Ed.), *Elderly patients and their doctors.* New York: Springer Publishing Company.

Marshall, G. N., Hays, R. D., Sherbourne, C. D., & Wells, K. B. (1993). The structure of patient satisfaction with outpatient medical care. *Psychological Assessment, 5*, 477–483.

Martin, D. P., Gilson, B. S., Bergner, M., Bobbitt, R. A., Pollard, W. E., Conn, J. R., & Cole, W. A. (1976). The Sickness Impact Profile: Potential use of a health status instrument for physician training. *Journal of Medical Education, 51*, 942–947.

Marvel, M. K., Epstein, R. M., Flowers, K., & Beckman, H. B. (1999). Soliciting the patient's agenda: Have we improved? *Journal of the American Medical Association, 281*, 283–287.

Maynard, C. L., Fisher, D., Passamani, E. R., & Pullum, T. (1986). Blacks in the Coronary Artery Surgery Study (CASS): Race and clinical decision making. *American Journal of Public Health, 76*, 1446–1448.

McGaghie, W. C. (2002). Assessing readiness for medical education: Evolution of the medical college admission test. *Journal of the American Medical Association, 288*, 1085–1090.

McKinlay, J. B. (1975). Who is really ignorant—Physician or patient? *Journal of Health and Social Behavior, 16*, 3–11.

McKinlay, J. B., Lin, T., Freund, K., & Moskowitz, M. (2002). The unexpected influence of physician attributes on clinical decisions: Results of an experiment. *Journal of Health and Social Behavior, 43*, 92–106.

McMahon, G. T. (2004). Coming to America: International medical graduates in the United States. *New England Journal of Medicine, 350*, 2435–2437.

McWhinney, I. (1989). The need for a transformed clinical method. In M. Stewart & D. Roter (Eds.), *Communicating with medical patients* (pp. 25–40). Newbury Park, CA: Sage.

Mead, N., & Bower, P. (2000). Patient-centredness: A conceptual framework and review of the empirical literature. *Social Science & Medicine, 55*, 283–299.

Mechanic, D. (1974). *Politics, medicine, and social science.* New York: John Wiley & Sons.

Mechanic, D. (1978). *Medical sociology*, 2nd ed. New York: The Free Press.

Mechanic, D., McAlpine, D. D., & Rosenthal, M. (2001). Are patients' office visits with physicians getting shorter? *New England Journal of Medicine, 344*, 198–204.

Miller, R. W. (1983). Doctors, patients don't communicate. *FDA Consumer.* HHS Publication No. (FDA) 83–1102.

Miller, S. M., & Mangan, C. E. (1983). Interacting effects of information and coping style in adapting to gynecologic stress: Should the doctor tell all? *Journal of Personality and Social Psychology, 45*, 223–236.

Mills, R. T., & Krantz, D. (1979). Information choice and reactions to stress: A field experiment in a blood bank with laboratory analogue. *Journal of Personality and Social Psychology, 37*, 608–620.

Milmoe, S., Rosenthal, R., Blane, H. T., Chafetz, M. E., & Wolf, I. (1967). The doctor's voice: Postdictor of successful referral of alcoholic patients. *Journal of Abnormal Psychology, 72*, 78–84.

Mishler, E. G. (1984). *The discourse of medicine: Dialectics of medical interviews.* Norwood, NJ: Ablex.

Mizrahi, T. (1986). *Getting rid of patients: Contradictions in the socialization of physicians.* New Brunswick, NJ: Rutgers University Press.

Morrell, D. C., Evans, M. E., & Morris, R. W. (1986). The "five-minute" consultation: Effect of time constraint on clinical content and patient satisfaction. *British Medical Journal, 292*, 870–872.

Morrison, G. (2005). Mortgaging our future: The cost of medical education. *New England Journal of Medicine, 352*, 117–119.

Mullen, P., van den Borne, B., & Breemhaar, B. (2000). Implementing a surgery-patient education program as a routine practice: A study conducted in two Dutch hospitals. *Patient Education and Counseling, 52*, 7–16.

Mumford, E., Schlesinger, H. J., & Glass, G. V. (1982). The effects of psychological intervention on recovery from surgery and heart attacks: An analysis of the literature. *American Journal of Public Health, 72*, 141–151.

Nielson-Bohlman, L., Panzer, A. M., & Kindig, D. A. (Eds). (2004). *Health literacy: A prescription to end confusion.* Committee on Health Literacy, Institute of Medicine, Washington, DC: National Academies Press.

Nordholm, L. A. (1980). Beautiful patients are good patients: Evidence for the physical attractiveness stereotype in first impressions of patients. *Social Science & Medicine, 14A*, 81–83.

Novack, D. H., Dube, C., & Goldstein, M. G. (1992). Teaching medical interviewing: A basic course on interviewing and the physician-patient relationship. *Archives of Internal Medicine, 152*, 1814–1820.

Oatley, K., & Jenkins, J. M. (1996). *Understanding emotions.* Cambridge, MA: Blackwell.

Ogden, J., Branson, R., Bryett, A., Campbell, A., Bebles, A., Ferguson, I., et al. (2003). What's in a name? An experimental study of patients' views of the impact and function of a diagnosis. *Family Practice, 20*, 248–253.

Ong, L. M. L., de Haes, J. C. J. M., Hoos, A. M., & Lammes, F. B. (1995). Doctor-patient communication: A review of the literature. *Social Science & Medicine, 40*, 903–918.

Ong, L. M. L., Visser, M. R. M., Lammes, F. B., & de Haes, J. C. J. M. (2000). Doctor-patient communication and cancer patients' quality of life and satisfaction. *Patient Education and Counseling, 41*, 145–156.

Orleans, C. T. (1985). Understanding and promoting smoking cessation: Overview and guidelines for physician intervention. *Annual Review of Medicine, 36*, 51–61.

Ornstein, S. M., Markert, G. P., Johnson, A. H., Rust, P. F., & Afrin, L. B. (1988). The effect of physician personality on laboratory test ordering for hypertensive patients. *Medical Care, 26*, 536–543.

Orth, J. E., Stiles, W. B., Scherwitz, L., Hennrikus, D., & Vallbona, C. (1987). Patient exposition and provider explanation in routine interviews and hypertensive patients' blood pressure control. *Health Psychology, 6*, 29–42.

Osler, W. (1903). On the need of a radical reform in our methods of teaching senior students. *Medical News, 82*, 49–53.

Osler, W. (1904). The master-word in medicine. In *Aequanimitas with other addresses to medical students, nurses, and practitioners of medicine.* Philadelphia: Blakiston.

Parikh, N. S., Parker, R. M., Nurss, J. R., Baker, D. W., & Williams, M. V. (1996). Shame and health literacy: The unspoken connection. *Patient Education and Counseling, 27*, 33–39.

Parsons, T. (1951). *The social system.* Glencoe, IL: The Free Press.

Parsons, T. (1975). The sick role and the role of the physician reconsidered. *Milbank Memorial Fund Quarterly, 53*, 257–278.

Patrick, C. J., Craig, K. D., & Prkachin, K. M. (1986). Observer judgments of acute pain: Facial action determinants. *Journal of Personality and Social Psychology, 50*, 1291–1298.

Pearse, W. H. (1994). The Commonwealth *Fund Women's Health Survey: Selected results and comments. Women's Health Issues, 4*, 38–47.

Pendleton, D. A., & Bochner, S. (1980). The communication of medical information in general practice consultations as a function of patients' social class. *Social Science & Medicine, 14A*, 669–673.

Pendleton, L., & House, W. C. (1984). Preferences for treatment approaches in medical care: College students versus diabetic outpatients. *Medical Care, 22*, 644–646.

Pfeiffer, C., Madray, H., Ardolino, A., & Willms, J. (1998). The rise and fall of students' skill in obtaining a medical history. *Medical Education, 32*, 283–288.

Philibert, I., Friedmann, P., & Williams, W. T. (2005). New requirements for resident duty hours. *Journal of the American Medical Association, 288,* 1112–1114.

Pickering, G. (1979). Therapeutics: Art or science? *Journal of the American Medical Association, 242*, 649–653.

Pratt, L., Seligmann, A., & Reader, G. (1957). Physicians' views on the level of medical information among patients. *American Journal of Public Health, 47*, 1277–1283.

President's Commission for the Study of Ethical Problems in Medicine and Biomedical and Behavioral Research. (1982). *Making health care decisions: The ethical and legal implications of informed consent in the patient-practitioner relationship.* Vol. 1. Washington, DC: Government Printing Office.

Price, J. H., Desmond, S. M., Snyder, F. F., & Kimmel, S. R. (1988). Perceptions of family practice residents regarding health care and poor patients. *Journal of Family Practice, 27*, 615–621.

Pringle, M., & Stewart-Evans, C. (1990). Does awareness of being video recorded affect doctors' consultation behavior? *British Journal of General Practice, 40*, 455–458.

Prkachin, K. M. (1992). Dissociating spontaneous and deliberate expressions of pain: Signal detection analyses. *Pain, 51*, 297–306.

Prohaska, T. R., & Glasser, M. (1996). Patients' views of family involvement in medical care decisions and encounters. *Research on Aging, 18*, 52–69.

Putnam, S. M., Stiles, W. B., Jacob, M. C., & James, S. A. (1988). Teaching the medical interview: An intervention study. *Journal of General Internal Medicine, 3*, 38–47.

Quine, L., & Pahl, J. (1986). First diagnosis of severe mental handicap: Characteristics of unsatisfactory encounters between doctors and parents. *Social Science & Medicine, 22*, 53–62.Quill, T. E. (1983). Partnerships in patient care: A contractual approach. *Annals of Internal Medicine, 98*, 228–234.

Quint, J. (1972). Institutionalized practices of information control. In E. Freidson & J. Lorber (Eds.), *Medical men and their work: A sociological reader.* Chicago: Aldine Atherton.

Rainey, L. C. (1985). Effects of preparatory patient education for radiation oncology patients. *Cancer, 56*, 1056–1061.

Ramirez, A. J., Graham, J., Richards, M. A., Cull, A., & Gregory, W. M. (1996). Mental health of hospital consultants: The effects of stress and satisfaction at work. *Lancet, 347*, 724–728.

Reader, G. S., Pratt, L., & Mudd, M. C. (1957). What do patients expect from their doctors? *Modern Hospital, 89*, 88–91.

Redman, S., Dickinson, J. A., Cockburn, J., Hennrikus, D., & Sanson-Fisher, R. W. (1989). The assessment of reactivity in direct observation studies of doctor-patient interactions. *Psychology and Health, 3*, 17–28.

Reeder, L. G. (1972). The patient-client as a consumer: Some observations on the changing professional-client relationship. *Journal of Health and Social Behavior, 13*, 406–412.

Rees, C., & Sheard, C. (2002). The relationship between medical students' attitudes towards communication skills learning and their demographic and education-related characteristics. *Medical Education, 36*, 1017–1027.

Reichardt, C. S., & Cook, T. D. (1969). *Qualitative and quantitative methods in evaluation research.* Beverly Hills, CA: Sage.

Ridsdale, L., Carruthers, M., Morris, R., & Ridsdale, J. (1989). Study of the effect of time availability on the consultation. *Journal of the Royal College of General Practice, 39*, 488–491.

Robinson, J. W., & Roter, D. L. (1999). Counseling by primary care physicians of patients who disclose psychosocial problems. *Journal of Family Practice, 48*, 698–705.

Rodin, J., & Langer, E. J. (1977). Long-term effects of a control-relevant intervention with the institutionalized aged. *Journal of Personality and Social Psychology, 35*, 897–902.

Rogoff, N. (1957). The decision to study medicine. In Merton, R. K., Reader, G. G., & Kendall, P. L. (Eds.), *The student-physician.* Cambridge, Massachusetts: Harvard University Press.

Rosenberg, E. L., Ekman, P., Jiang, W., Babyak, M., Coleman, R. E., Hanson, M., O'Connor, C., et al. (2001). Linkages between facial expressions of anger and transient myocardial ischemia in men with coronary artery disease. *Emotion, 1*, 107–115.

Rosenthal, R., & Rosnow, R. L. (1991). *Essentials of behavioral research: Methods and data analysis,* 2nd ed. New York: McGraw-Hill.

Ross, C. E., & Duff, R. S. (1982). Returning to the doctor: The effects of client characteristics, type of practice, and experiences with care. *Journal of Health and Social Behavior, 23*, 119–131.

Ross, C. E., Mirowsky, J., & Duff, R. S. (1982). Physician status characteristics and client satisfaction in two types of medical practice. *Journal of Health and Social Behavior, 23*, 317.

Ross, S. E., & Lin, C-T. (2003). The effects of promoting patient access to medical records: A review. *Journal of the American Medical Informatics Association, 10*, 129–139.

Roter, D. L. (1977). Patient participation in the patient-provider interaction: The effects of patient question asking on the quality of interaction, satisfaction, and compliance. *Health Education Monographs, 5*, 281–315.

Roter, D. L. (1991). Elderly patient-physician communication: A descriptive study of content and affect during the medical encounter. *Advances in Health Education, 3*, 15–23.

Roter, D. L. (2000a). The outpatient medical encounter and elderly patients. *Clinics in Geriatric Medicine, 16*, 95–107.

Roter, D. L. (2000b). The enduring and evolving nature of the patient-physician relationship. *Patient Education and Counseling, 39*, 5–15.

Roter, D. L. (2004). Health literacy and the patient provider relationship. In J. Schwartzberg, J. Van Geest, C. Wang, J. Gazmararian, R. Parker, D. Roter, R. Rudd, & D. Schillinger (Eds.), *Understanding health literacy: Implications for medicine and public health.* Chicago, IL: AMA Press.

Roter, D. L., Erby, H. L., Larson S., McDonald, E., Cho, J. H., & Ellington, L. (2006). Assessing oral literacy burden of genetic counseling dialogue. Unpublished manuscript, The Johns Hopkins University.

Roter, D. L., & Frankel, R. (1992). Quantitative and qualitative approaches to the evaluation of the medical dialogue. *Social Science & Medicine, 34*, 1097–1103.

Roter, D. L., Geller, G., Bernhardt, B. A., Larson, S. M., & Doksum, T. (1999). Effects of obstetrician gender on communication and patient satisfaction. *Obstetrics and Gynecology, 93*, 635–641.

Roter, D. L., & Hall, J. A. (1987). Physicians' interviewing styles and medical information obtained from patients. *Journal of General Internal Medicine, 2*, 325–329.

Roter, D. L., & Hall, J. A. (2004). Physician gender and patient-centered communication: A critical review of empirical research. *Annual Review of Public Health, 25*, 497–519.

Roter, D. L., Hall, J. A., & Aoki, Y. (2002). Physician gender effects in medical communication: A meta-analytic review. *Journal of the American Medical Association, 288*, 756–764.

Roter, D. L., Hall, J. A., & Katz, N. R. (1987). Relations between physicians' behaviors and analogue patients' satisfaction, recall, and impressions. *Medical Care, 25*, 437–451.

Roter, D. L., Hall, J. A., & Katz, N. R. (1988). Patient-physician communication: A descriptive review of the literature. *Patient Education and Counseling, 12*, 99–119.

Roter, D. L., Hall, J. A., Kern, D. E., Barker, L. R., Cole, K. A., & Roca, R. P. (1995). Improving physicians' interviewing skills and reducing patients' emotional distress: A randomized clinical trial. *Archives of Internal Medicine, 155*, 1877–1884.

Roter, D. L., Hall, J. A., Merisca, R., Ruehle, B., Cretin, D., & Svarstad, B. (1998). Effectiveness of interventions to improve patient compliance: A meta-analysis. *Medical Care, 36*, 1138–1161.

Roter, D. L., Larson, S., Fischer, C. S., Arnold, R. M., & Tulsky, J. A. (2000). Experts practice what they preach: A descriptive study of best and normative practices in end of life discussions. *Archives of Internal Medicine, 160*, 3477–3485.

Roter, D. L., Larson, S., Sands, D., Ford, D., & Houston, T. (2006). Can e-mail messages between patients and physicians be patient-centered? *Health Communication,* forthcoming.

Roter, D. L., Lipkin, M., Jr., & Korsgaard, A. (1991). Sex differences in patients' and physicians' communication during primary care medical visits. *Medical Care, 29*, 1083–1093.

Roter, D. L., Stewart, M., Putnam, S., Lipkin, M., Stiles, W., & Inui, T. (1997). Communication patterns of primary care physicians. *Journal of the American Medical Association, 270*, 350–355.

Roter, D. L., & McNeilis, K. S. (2003). The nature of the therapeutic relationship and the assessment and consequences of its discourse in routine medical visits. In T. Thompson, A. Dorsey, K. Miller, & R. Parrott (Eds.), *Handbook of health communication.* Mahwah, NJ: Lawrence Erlbaum Associates.

Roth, J. A. (1963). Information and the control of treatment in tuberculosis hospitals. In E. Freidson (Ed.), *The hospital in modern society.* London: Free Press of Glencoe.

Rubenstein, L. Z., Schairer, C., Wieland, G. D., & Kane, R. (1984). Systematic biases in functional status assessment of elderly adults: Effects of different data sources. *Journal of Gerontology, 39,* 686–691.

Russell, N. K., & Roter, D. L. (1993). Discussion of lifestyle topics in primary care medical visits. *American Journal of Public Health, 83,* 979–982.

Sacks, H., Schegloff, E. A., & Jefferson, G. (1974). A simplest systematic for the organization of turn-taking for conversation. *Language, 50,* 696–735.

Saha, S., Komaromy, M., Koepsell, T. D., & Bindman, A. B. (1999). Patient-physician racial concordance and the perceived quality and use of health care. *Archives of Internal Medicine, 159,* 997–1004.

Sala, F., Krupat, E., & Roter, D. (2002). Satisfaction and the use of humor by physicians and patients. *Psychology and Health, 17,* 269–280.

Santo, A., Laizner, A. M., & Shohet, L. (2005). Exploring the value of audiotapes for health literacy: A systematic review. *Patient Education and Counseling, 58,* 235–243.

Sarason, B. R., Sarason, I. G., Hacker, T. A., & Basham, R. B. (1985). Concomitants of social support: Social skills, physical attractiveness, and gender. *Journal of Personality and Social Psychology, 49,* 469–480.

Schilling, L. M., Scatena, L., Steiner, J. F., Albertson, G. A., Lin, C. T., Cyran, L., et al. (2002). The third person in the room: Frequency, role, and influence of companions during primary care medical encounters. *Journal of Family Practice, 51,* 685–690.

Schillinger, D., Bindman, A. B., Wang, F., Stewart, A., & Piette, J. (2004). Functional health literacy and the quality of physician-patient communication among diabetes patients. *Patient Education and Counseling, 52,* 315-23.

Schillinger, D., Piette, J., Grumbach, K., Wang, F., Wilson, C., Daher, C., et al. (2003). Closing the loop: Physician communication with diabetic patients who have low health literacy. *Archives of Internal Medicine, 163,* 83–90.

Schmitt, F. E., & Woolridge, P. J. (1973). Psychological preparation of surgical patients. *Nursing Research, 22,* 108–116.

Schmittdiel, J., Grumback, K., Selby, J. V., & Quesenberry, C. P. (2000). Effect of physician and patient gender concordance on patient satisfaction and preventive care practices. *Journal of General Internal Medicine, 5,* 761–769.

Schneider, C. E. (1998). *The practice of autonomy: Patients, doctors, and medical decisions.* New York: Oxford University Press.

Schulman, K. A., Berlin, J. A., Harless, W., Kerner, J. F., Sistrunk, S., & Gersh, B. J. (1999). The effect of race and sex on physicians' recommendations for cardiac catheterization. *New England Journal of Medicine, 340,* 618–626.

Shafer, A., Reflections of a part-time physician. *Academic Medicine, 79,* 357.

Shapiro, D. E., Boggs, S. R., Melamed, B. G., & Graham-Pole, J. (1992). The effects of varied physician affect on recall, anxiety, and perceptions in women at risk for breast cancer: An analogue study. *Health Psychology, 11*, 61–66.

Shenkin, B., & Warner, D. (1973). Giving the patient his medical record: A proposal to improve the system. *New England Journal of Medicine, 289*, 688–691.

Shorter, E. (1985). *Bedside manners.* New York: Simon and Schuster.

Skipper, J. K., Tagliacozzo, D. L., & Mauksch, H. O. (1964). Some possible consequences of limited communication between patients and hospital functionaires. *Journal of Health and Human Behavior, 6*, 34–39.

Smedley, B. D., Stith, A. Y., & Nelson, A. R. (Eds). (2003). *Unequal treatment: Confronting racial and ethnic disparities in health care.* Committee on Understanding and Eliminating Racial and Ethnic Disparities in Health Care, Institute of Medicine. Washington, DC: National Academies Press.

Smith, R. C., & Zimny, G. H. (1988). Physicians' emotional reactions to patients. *Psychosomatics, 29*, 392–397.

Smith, R. C., Marshall-Dorsey, A. A., Osborn, G. G., Shebroe, V., Lyles, J. S., Stoffelmayr, B. E., et al. (2000). Evidence-based guidelines for teaching patient-centered interviewing. *Patient Education and Counseling, 39*, 27–36.

Speedling, E. J., & Rose, D. N. (1985). Building an effective doctor-patient relationship: From patient satisfaction to patient participation. *Social Science & Medicine, 21*, 115–120.

Stafford, R. S., Saglam, D., Causino, N., Starfield, B., Culpepper, L., Marder, W. D., & Blumenthal, D. (1999). Trends in adult visits to primary care physicians in the United States. *Archives of Family Medicine, 8*, 26–32.

Starfield, B., Wray, C., Hess, K., Gross, R., Birk, P. S., & D'Lugoff, B. C. (1981). The influence of patient-practitioner agreement on outcome of care. *American Journal of Public Health, 71*, 127–131.

Steptoe, A., Sutcliffe, I., Allen, B., & Coombes, C. (1991). Satisfaction with communication, medical knowledge, and coping style in patients with metastatic cancer. *Social Science & Medicine, 32*, 627–632.

Stewart, M. A. (1983). Patient characteristics which are related to the doctor-patient interaction. *Family Practice, 1*, 30–35.

Stewart, M. A. (1984). What is a successful doctor-patient interview? A study of interactions and outcomes. *Social Science & Medicine, 19*, 167–175.

Stewart, M. A. (1995). Effective physician-patient communication and health outcomes: A review. *Canadian Medical Association Journal, 152*, 1423–1433.

Stewart, M. A., Brown, B. J., Weston, W. W., McWhinney, I., McWilliam, C. L., & Freeman, T. R. (Eds.). (1995). *Patient-centered medicine: Transforming the clinical method.* Thousand Oaks, CA: Sage.

Stiles, W. B. (1992). *Describing talk: A taxonomy of verbal response modes.* Newbury Park, CA: Sage.

Stilwell, N. A., Wallick, M. M., Thal, S. E., & Burleson, J. A. (2000). Myers-Briggs type and medical specialty choice: A new look at an old question. *Teaching and Learning in Medicine, 12*, 14–20.

Stoeckle, J. D., & Barsky, A. (1981). Attributions: Uses of social science knowledge in doctoring in primary care. In L. Eisenberg & A. Kleinman (Eds.), *The relevance of social science for medicine.* Boston: D. Reidel.

Strasser, F., Fisch, M., Bodurka, D. C., Sivesind, D., & Bruera, E. (2002). E-emotions: Email for written emotional expression. *Journal of Clinical Oncology, 20,* 3352–3355.

Stratton, T. D., McLaughlin, M. A., Witte, F. M., Fosson, S. E., & Nora, L. M. (2005). Does students' exposure to gender discrimination and sexual harassment in medical school affect specialty choice and residency program selection? *Academic Medicine, 80,* 400–408.

Street, R. L., Jr., & Buller, D. B. (1987). Nonverbal response patterns in physician-patient interactions: A functional analysis. *Journal of Nonverbal Behavior, 11,* 234–253.

Street, R. L., Jr., & Buller, D. B. (1988). Patients' characteristics affecting physician-patient nonverbal communication. *Human Communication Research, 15,* 60–90.

Strull, W. M., Lo, B., & Charles, G. (1984). Do patients want to participate in medical decision making? *Journal of the American Medical Association, 252,* 2990–2994.

Studdert, D. M., Mello, M. M., Sage, W. M., DesRoches, C. M., Peugh, J., Zapert, K., et al. (2005). Defensive medicine among high-risk specialist physicians in a volatile malpractice environment. *Journal of the American Medical Association, 293,* 2609–2617.

Suchman, A. L, Roter, D. L., Greene, M., & Lipkin, M., Jr. (1993). Physician satisfaction with primary care office visits. *Medical Care, 31,* 1083–1092.

Svarstad, B. L. (1974). *The doctor-patient encounter: An observational study of communication and outcome.* Doctoral dissertation, Department of Sociology, University of Wisconsin, Madison, Wisconsin.

Szasz, P. S., & Hollender, M. H. (1956). A contribution to the philosophy of medicine: The basic model of the doctor-patient relationship. *Archives of Internal Medicine, 97,* 585–592.

Thibault, G. E. (1997). Bedside rounds revisited. *New England Journal of Medicine, 336,* 1174–1175.

Thompson, T. L. (1994). Interpersonal communication and health care. In M. L. Knapp & G. R. Miller (Eds.), *Handbook of interpersonal communication,* 2nd ed. (pp. 696–725). Thousand Oaks, CA: Sage.

Thompson, S. C., Nanni, C., & Schwankovsky, L. (1990). Patient-oriented interventions to improve communication in a medical office visit. *Health Psychology, 9,* 390–404.

Tresolini, C. P., and the Pew-Fetzer Task Force on Advancing Psychosocial Health Education. (1994). *Health professions education and relationship-centered care.* San Francisco: Pew Health Professions Commission.

Tuckett, D., Boulton, M., Olson, C., & Williams, A. (1985). *Meetings between experts.* New York: Tavistock Publications.

U.S. Department of Health and Human Services (1999). *Mental health: A report of the Surgeon General.* Rockville, MD: U.S. Department of Health and Human Services.

Van den Brink-Muinen, A., van Dulmen, S., Messerli-Rohrbach, V., & Bensing, J. (2002). Do gender dyads have different communication patterns? A comparative study in Western-European general practices. *Patient Education and Counseling, 48,* 253–264.

Van den Brink-Muinen, A., Verhaak, P. F. M., & Bensing, J. M. (1999). *The Euro-communication Study.* Utrecht: NIVEL.

van Ryn, M. (2002). Research on the provider contribution to race/ethnicity disparities in medical care. *Medical Care, 40,* Supplement, I140–I151.

Van Wieringen, J. C., Harmsen, J. A., Brujnzeels, M. A. (2002). Intercultural communication in general practice. *European Journal of Public Health, 12,* 63–68.

Veasey, S., Rosen, R., Barzansky, B., Rosen, I., & Owens, J. (2002). Sleep loss and fatigue in residency training: A reappraisal. *Journal of the American Medical Association, 288,* 1116–1124.

Verbrugge, L. M., & Steiner, R. P. (1981). Physician treatment of men and women patients: Sex bias or appropriate care? *Medical Care, 19,* 609–632.

Verghese, A. (March 16, 2003). Hard Cures. *New York Times,* Sunday Magazine Section, pp. 11–12.

Vertinsky, I. B., Thompson, W. A., & Uyeno, D. (1974). Measuring consumer desire for participation in clinical decision making. *Health Services Research, 9,* 121–134.

Waitzkin, H. (1985). Information-giving in medical care. *Journal of Health and Social Behavior, 26,* 81–101.

Wallen, J., Waitzkin, H., & Stoeckle, J. D. (1979). Physician stereotypes about female health and illness. *Women & Health, 4,* 135–146.

Wasserman, R. C., Inui, T. S., Barriatua, R. D., Carter, W. B., & Lippincott, P. (1983). Responsiveness to maternal concern in preventive child health visits: An analysis of clinician-parent interactions. *Developmental and Behavioral Pediatrics, 4,* 171–176.

Weisman, C. S., & Teitelbaum, M. A. (1989). Women and health care communication. *Patient Education and Counseling, 13,* 183–199.

Whelan, G. P., Gary, N. E., Kostis, J., Boulet, J. R., & Hallock, J. A. (2002). The changing pool of international medical graduates seeking certification training in U.S. graduate medical education programs. *Journal of the American Medical Association, 288,* 1079–1084.

Whelan, G. P., McKinley, D. W., Boulet, J. R., Macrae, J., & Kamholz, S. (2001). Validation of the doctor-patient communication component of the Educational Commission for Foreign Medical Graduates Clinical Skills Assessment. *Medical Education, 45*, 757–761.

White, C. B., Moyer, C. A., Stern, D. T., & Katz, S. J. (2004). A content analysis of e-mail communication between patients and their providers: Patients get the message. *Journal of the American Medical Informatics Association, 11*, 260–267.

White, J., Levinson, W., & Roter, D. (1994). "Oh, by the way . . .": The closing moments of the medical visit. *Journal of General Internal Medicine, 9*, 24–28.

White, K. L. (1988). *The task of medicine: Dialogue at Wickenburg.* Menlo Park, California: The Henry J. Kaiser Family Foundation.

Whitney, S. N., Brown, B. W., Brody, H., Alcser, K. H., Bachman, J. G., & Greely, H. T. (2001). Views of United States physicians and members of the American Medical Association *House of Delegates on physician-assisted suicide. Journal of General Internal Medicine, 16*, 290–296.

Williams, G. C., & Deci, E. L. (1996). Internalization of biopsychosocial values by medical students: a test of self-determination theory. *Journal of Personality and Social Psychology, 70*, 767–779.

Williams, J. G., Cheung, W-Y, Chetwynd, N., Cohen, D. R., El-Sharkawi, S., Finlay, I., et al. (2001). Pragmatic randomized trial to evaluate the use of patient held records for the continuing care of patients with cancer. *Quality in Health Care, 10*, 159–165.

Williams, M. V., Baker, D. W., Parker, R. M., & Nurss, J. R. (1998). Relationship of functional health literacy to patients' knowledge of their chronic disease: A study of patients with hypertension and diabetes. *Archives of Internal Medicine, 158*, 166–72.

Williams, S., Weinman, J., & Dale, J. (1998). Doctor-patient communication and patient satisfaction: A review. *Family Practice, 15*, 480–92.

Willson, P., & McNamara, J. R. (1982). How perceptions of a simulated physician-patient interaction influence intended satisfaction and compliance. *Social Science & Medicine, 16*, 1699–1703.

Wilson, A. D. (1985). Consultation length: General practitioners' attitudes and practices. *British Medical Journal, 290*, 1322–1324. Wilson, A. D., McDonald, P., Hayes, L., & Cooney, J. (1992). Health promotion in the general practice consultation: A minute makes a difference. *British Medical Journal, 304*, 227–234.

Woloschuk, W., Harasym, P. H., & Temple, W. (2004). Attitude change during medical school: A cohort study. *Medical Education, 48*, 522–534.

Xu, G., Fields, S. K., Laine, C., Veloski, J. J., Barzansky, B., Marini, C. J. (1997). The relationship between the race/ethnicity of generalist physicians and their care for underserved populations. *American Journal of Public Health, 87*, 817–822.

Yager, J., & Linn, L. S. (1981). Physician-patient agreement about depression: Notation in medical records. *General Hospital Psychiatry, 3*, 271–276.

Zborowski, M. (1952). Cultural components in responses to pain. *Journal of Social Issues, 4*, 16–30.

Zola, I. K. (1963). Problems of communication, diagnosis, and patient care: The interplay of patient, physician and clinic organization. *Journal of Medical Education, 38*, 829–838.

Zola, I. K. (1966). Culture and symptoms: An analysis of patients' presenting complaints. *American Sociological Review, 31*, 615–630.

Subject Index

Author Index

About the Authors

DEBRA L. ROTER holds joint appointments as Professor of Health, Behavior and Society at the Johns Hopkins Bloomberg School of Public Health and the Johns Hopkins Schools of Medicine and Nursing.

JUDITH A. HALL is Professor of Psychology at Northeastern University.